Using Drama with Children on the Autism Spectrum

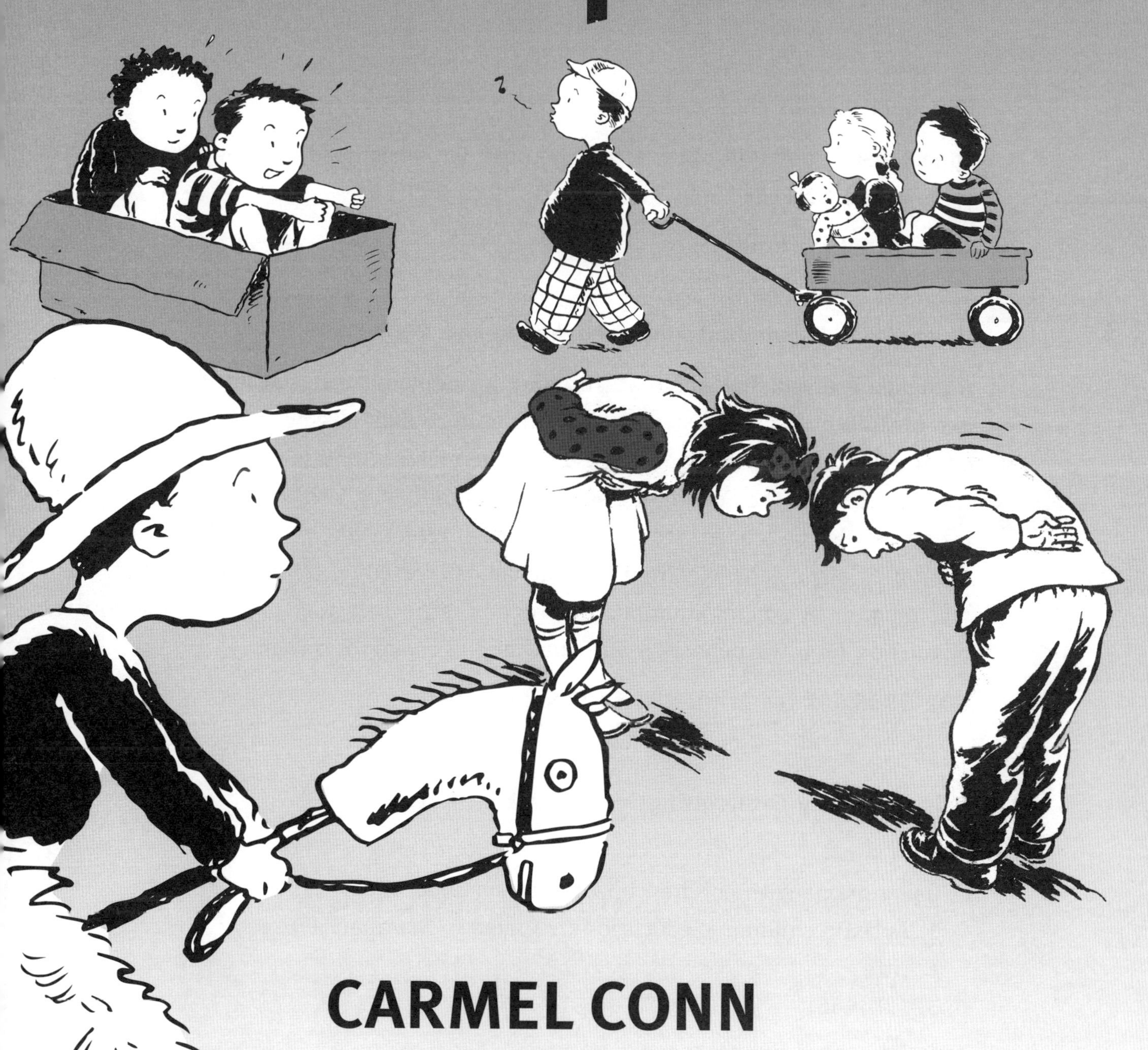

Using Drama with Children on the Autism Spectrum

CARMEL CONN

Speechmark

First published in 2007 by

Speechmark Publishing Ltd, 8 Oxford Court, St James Road, Brackley NN13 7XY, UK
Tel: +44 (0) 1280 845 570 Fax: +44 (0) 1280 845 584

www.speechmark.net

© Carmel Conn, 2007
Illustrations © Jane Bottomley and Woody Fox, 2007

002-5366/Printed in the United Kingdom/1010

British Library Cataloguing in Publication Data

Conn, Carmel
    Using drama with children on the autism spectrum
    1. Autistic children – Education 2. Drama – Therapeutic use
    I. Title
    371.9'4466
ISBN-13: 978 0 86388 601 0

Contents

List of Activities

5 Props, Puppets, Costume *Exploring objects and people as objects*

6 Me, Myself, I *Exploring aspects of the self*

7 Storytelling *Recalling events/making meaning*

List of Assessments

Acknowledgements

The content of this book is the result of many hours playing and interacting with children, and learning from them. The author would like to thank the children, parents and staff with whom she has worked over the years. In particular, she is indebted to Cheryl Roberts for her examples of scripts, to Claire Hayes and Sharon Carpentier for their thoughts on working with feelings, and to Nataly Fernandes for her anecdote about her son. Thanks too to Cath Conn and Glynis Thomas for reading first drafts of the book.

This book is for Phyllis, and for Osian of course.

Preface

For children with autism, who have difficulty in understanding and engaging with ordinary social interaction as it happens, drama provides a safe and structured way of first watching and then engaging with other people. The aim of this book is to make the case for drama as an effective way of working with primary age children on the autism spectrum. *Using Drama with Children on the Autism Spectrum* contains over 150 drama games and activities to promote skills in:

- social understanding
- social communication
- expression and play.

It is intended to be read as a whole with ideas on how to work with children developed across the units of the book. However, it is possible to use units discretely, commencing work at any point in the book depending on the needs of the child. Each unit is designed to focus on one skill at a time, addressing areas such as mirroring, emotional expression and pretence, which are commonly difficult for children with autism. Advice is provided on assessment and planning so that practitioners can establish where to begin work with a child.

Using Drama with Children on the Autism Spectrum promotes the idea of working in inclusive groups of children, with and without autism, where the child with autism can learn from the models provided by others who, in turn, can be taught how to be more effective in their responses and more aware of what autism is.

As an experienced teacher and therapist who has worked with a large number of children with autism in a wide variety of educational settings and across the age range, I am aware that no two children with autism are alike. Children respond in different ways to the same approach and can develop to very different degrees in terms of their social communication. *Using Drama with Children on the Autism Spectrum* includes a range of activities, which may be too difficult for some children but very enjoyable to others. However, the underlying premise of all activities in the book is that work on developing social communication and understanding in children with autism should be carefully structured, with opportunity provided for appropriate levels of support.

Using Drama with Children on the Autism Spectrum is designed for use with children aged between 5 and 11 years old. It takes a developmental approach with Part I focusing on the preverbal child, of any age, who is at an early stage of engagement, and Part II concentrating on higher level group work with more able children. The organisation of the two parts differs slightly in that Part I is more a general discussion of ways to provide stimulation and of interacting that are essentially drama-based, whilst Part II concerns specific programmes of work to develop personal and social skills using classic drama techniques.

Using Drama with Children on the Autism Spectrum includes the following:

- drama activities matched to areas of skill in social interaction, communication and play
- step-by-step guidance on how to deliver a drama programme
- support materials for activities
- developmental assessment profiles
- advice on target setting, planning, ways of working, setting up a group and useful resources.

I hope that the book will be of benefit to teachers, therapists and parents who are looking for new ways of engaging and working with children with autism and who are interested in the creative potential that drama provides.

Carmel Conn, 2007

How to use this book

Using Drama with Children on the Autism Spectrum is for use by mainstream teachers working with an included child with autism in primary school settings as well as teachers in special schools, advisory teachers, speech & language therapists, drama teachers and dramatherapists. Parents and other professionals involved with autism who are looking for ideas on how to develop language and communication, social understanding and play, may also be interested in the book.

The book is divided into two parts. The simple child-focused activities in Part I reflect what can be provided in a special school setting for a child with severe and complex needs. The emphasis in Part II, on mixed groups of children with and without autism, reflects what is available in included mainstream school placements, typically available to a child who has more verbal skill and social awareness or who has Asperger Syndrome.

Each unit of the book follows a similar format, but the work involved does become progressively harder. Children with autism are able to do only one thing at a time, and initial activities are broken down, wherever possible, into straightforward single skills. Later units require more in the way of a combination of skills learned in earlier units. The length of time spent on each unit of work depends on the needs of the child, but the general advice is that activities are repeated regularly to develop spontaneity, fluency, creativity and playfulness. Throughout the book, there is advice on how to use structure and gradually build a child's capacity for the target skills. Each unit contains:

- a brief theoretical background to the skill area which is the focus of the unit
- a clear set of aims
- an assessment profile
- a set of drama activities to develop the focus skill
- clear instructions for each activity, including the preparation and materials needed, if any
- general comments and advice on ways of working as well as specific suggestions for varying or extending activities.

Case study 'Snapshots' are also provided throughout the book, drawing on the author's own experience and work with children with autism. These Snapshots are included to help illustrate through practical example some aspects of the theoretical discussion.

At the end of the book, the Appendices provide photocopiable resources to support some of the activities and a list of useful contacts.

PART I Child-focused Work Relating through Drama

Part I outlines drama-based ways of stimulating and engaging a preverbal and withdrawn child. It is not intended for use as a discrete programme, but is more in the way of general advice on how to work through drama at this level. Activities would be used in conjunction with an overall approach that is based on interaction. The areas of work covered in Part I are:

1 An Empty Space *Working with the sensory environment*

Following models of interaction based on the intuitive reciprocal exchange of parent and infant, activities using the visual, aesthetic and sensory experience of drama are provided as a stimulus and basis for one-to-one interaction with a preverbal child with autism.

2 Simple Groups *Noticing others*

Focusing in particular on the repetition and ritual of simple activities that group work allows, activities are suggested for developing noticing and participatory behaviours in a child with autism.

PART II Group Work Building skills

The work of Part II is more programme-based with clear outlines of work that can be followed as a discrete area of learning over a series of drama sessions. However, it is also possible to dip into this part and select individual activities to support ongoing work on play, language and social communication, self-esteem, social skill and literacy. The areas of work that are covered in Part II are:

3 Sculpting *Using the body/starting to pretend*

By using simple activities to develop the use of the body and capacity for physical expression, a child with autism learns skills in play, pretence and social understanding.

4 **Scripts** *Rehearsing lines/encouraging speech*

Activities to promote speech through the development of vocal expression and the use of scripts, rehearsal and role play.

5 **Props, Puppets, Costume** *Exploring objects and people as objects*

Focuses on the fascination with objects of a child with autism and reflects on his experience that people are objects too. Activities aim to develop the child's ability to generalise his understanding of objects beyond a single narrow meaning.

6 **Me, Myself, I** *Exploring aspects of the self*

In autism, work on awareness of self and others is critical, development here bringing about an improvement in self-esteem and ability to function in social situations.

7 **Storytelling** *Recalling events/making meaning*

Activities to develop a child's understanding of narrative, enabling him to recall, make sense of and retell stories and lived experience.

8 **Improvisation** *Putting experience and emotion together*

How to use skills in improvisation, spontaneity and creativity to gain a better understanding of ordinary social experiences.

9 **Ending** *Working with the concept of 'finished'*

Highlights the importance of working with the concept of 'finished' for children with autism and provides suggestions for ending groups.

Assessment

There is an assessment profile linked to each unit. Profiles are designed for both formative assessment, to gauge what skills a child has, and summative assessment to record the child's response to the drama intervention at the end of a series of sessions. Areas of need identified by the profile can be addressed through use of the relevant activities in the section that follows.

Establishing starting levels

Units of work do not necessarily correspond to age and are based more on the developmental level of a child. Part I is likely to be the starting point for preverbal children as well as for children in the early years. Part II is for children who have some skills in language and interaction, with activities requiring increasing amounts of skill and understanding. Which unit to choose will be informed by the child's present identified individual needs and may support other ongoing targets.

Planning and record keeping

Each unit has a clear set of aims that reflect typical targets for a child with autism. Planning is aided in the way that units are set out, with activities grouped under different areas of work. Each area of work builds on the previous one so that units, like the book itself, take a developmental line.

Assessment profiles may be kept as part of a child's ongoing record of achievement. They can be regularly updated, with dates entered for when a particular skill was demonstrated by the child within a session and generalised beyond.

Symbols used in the book

The following symbol system is used in the book to provide additional information about activities:

1–3 This is used where activities follow a set sequence. The numbers indicate how many of the activities that follow are included in the sequence.

P This symbol is used where an activity is supported by the photocopiable resource materials which can be found in Appendix I at the back of the book.

8+ This symbol denotes that a large group, of at least eight, is needed for the activity. Please note that in the later units, particularly in Unit 8, there is a greater requirement for large groups of children.

↑ This symbol is used in Unit 2 to indicate where a higher level of adult support is needed to carry out group work.

Introduction

I am often surprised by the extent to which children who have a diagnosis of autism are able to participate in and really enjoy drama. Drama is specifically social and communicative in its method, concerned with verbal and non-verbal expression, pretence, creative thinking and empathy; in other words, all the things with which children with autism have difficulty. Not surprisingly, little is written about drama as an approach with autism. Yet from my experience of working with children in schools, drama sessions can have a great deal to offer.

This book will argue that drama can be used at every level of development to promote self-awareness and social skill in a child with autism. Drama is suitable for more able children, using role play, storytelling and improvisation to explore personal and social issues. It is also of benefit to preverbal children at the early stages of engagement, to encourage language, communication and social interaction. With its focus on 'life as art', drama provides a way of presenting life experiences in small digestible chunks with which a child with autism can more easily engage.

Essentially, drama concerns the individual in relation to people and to the world around, but can be considerably adapted in the way it is used. Relating to others can mean anything, from improvising in a group to interacting with one other person in one-to-one activity. Similarly, relating to the world around covers a sophisticated relating to a created imaginary world as well as simply responding to stimuli within the immediate environment. The adaptability of drama suits the fact that children with autism are different. Children with autism differ in how much language they have, in their level of interest in others, in the manner of their communication, in what they can imagine and in how creative they can be. Drama can be used in different ways to engage the child at whatever level he is at.

Why drama?

The following 'Snapshots' are examples of how drama can have a profound impact on children with autism.

The presence of others, always a feature of drama, can also act as a stimulus.

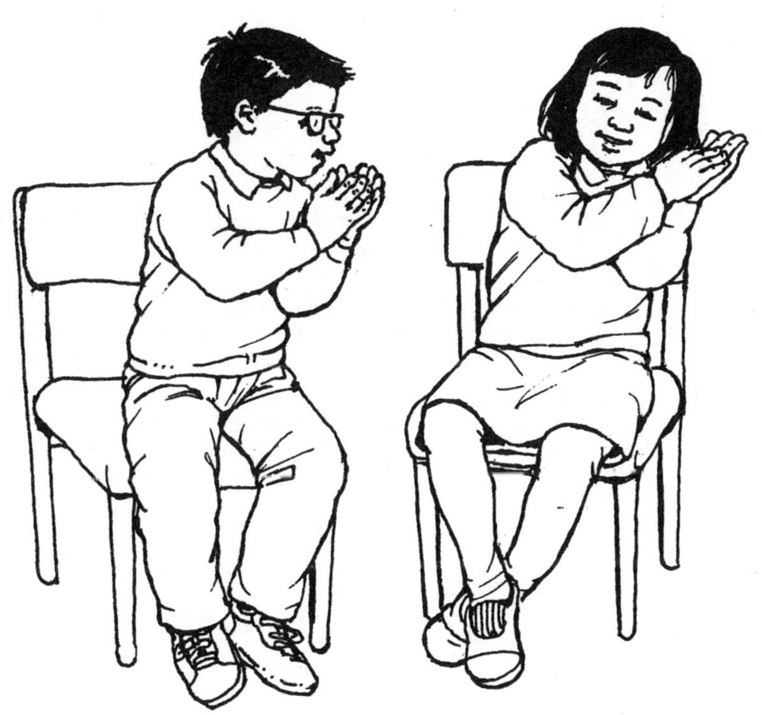

Drama allows real life to be practised in a setting that is safe, the artificiality of which appeals to someone for whom life itself may feel unreal.

⊙ snapshot _Owen_

Owen, aged ten, found it hard to know what to say to friends when engaged in conversation. In weekly drama workshops he practised using his voice, which was very soft, along with scripted lines of what he might say on given topics. He took part in role-played scenes with other children, exchanging lines from an agreed script. Drama games were used to play with the lines and encourage more expression and spontaneity in communication. The drama work was carried over into everyday life by Owen learning set lines and being prompted to use them by his support worker, other staff and peers who had been primed to support him in this way.

Creative drama and people with special needs

The use of drama as a means of helping people with various special needs in educational and community settings is well established. In such settings, drama work tends to be less a basis for performance and more an end in itself, a process that encourages creative expression and self-awareness. Quite often, the emphasis is on training: in social skills, group skills and skills of physical expression. Methods used include such things as body awareness and the use of all five senses, drama workshop games, improvisation, storytelling and role play. Scripted pieces may be used, but this is less common (Emunah, 1994).

Drama used in this way aims to develop personal understanding, ability and a sense of well-being, and is usually known as therapeutic or creative drama (Jennings, 1986; Chesner, 1998). The material for creative expression is from the client group's own experiences and lives. Indeed, it could be said that the drama work is partly about developing the client's ability to tap into his 'latent creative possibilities' (Jones, 1996).

Drama and autism

The idea of using creative drama with children with autism at first seems inappropriate. With autism, rarely can it be said that creativity is merely latent. The nature of the disorder and its effect on development means that the potential for creativity – for imaginative thought connected to real-life experience – is itself impaired. Autism implies an inability to make imaginative connections between things or with people, to understand cause and effect and, lacking a theory of mind, the minds of others (Baron-Cohen, 1995). Drama concerns the form and feeling of lived experience, but people with autism have difficulties processing and understanding social and emotional situations. Drama reflects on the self as it is experienced in the world and in relation to other people but, as Powell & Jordan (1993) point out, the inability to develop an 'experiencing self' and create self-narratives is a defining feature of autism.

Yet it is clearly the case that drama concerns itself with much that is at issue in autism. Interaction using verbal and non-verbal communication, self-expression and flexibility of expression, pretence and the creation of representative worlds, putting oneself in another's shoes and understanding other viewpoints, are typical aspects of any drama programme. They reflect what is impaired in autism, expressed by Wing & Gould (1979) as the triad of impairments:

- impairment of social interaction
- impairment of social communication
- impairment of social imagination and flexibility of thought.

Sue Jennings (1986) points out that an important aspect of creative drama is the practising of 'tasks and skills', developing a greater capacity for the skills needed to take part in everyday life. For children with autism, drama can be instrumental in allowing them to develop skills of interaction, social communication and imaginative thinking.

Drama can develop physical expression and understanding, the use of the body, the face and the voice in interaction. It can be used to build a capacity for pretence and all that implies in terms of reflecting on, defining and representing lived experiences. Interrelatedness and playfulness can be encouraged as part of the group work that drama ordinarily involves. Children are encouraged to learn skills in taking turns, sequencing and making stories together. Role play is used as a way of exploring 'Who am I?' as well as the role relationships commonly experienced in life: parent/child, teacher/pupil, friends. Above all, drama promotes the act of watching. Human interaction can be observed as it is happening and in a way that can be manipulated to see the nuances of what really goes on when two people communicate.

Given its potential to develop social-cognitive functioning, it is unsurprising that Gillberg (2004) gives drama as an effective form of working with children with autism second only to structured teaching.

Autism and learning

Powell (2000) has outlined two possible learning environments for the student with autism, the social and the asocial. The social learning environment replicates the pedagogy of the ordinary classroom where the teacher interacts continually with the pupils, teaching is language based and creative thinking is encouraged. Asocial learning differs in that the teacher is expected to operate more in an 'autistic environment'. Personal communication is kept to a minimum, lessons are clearly structured by some visual, non-verbal means and tasks are concrete. The emphasis of asocial learning is on getting the learning environment right rather than trying to change the learning make-up of the individual himself.

However, as Nind (2000) has argued, the response to a child with autism who thinks and interacts in an autistic way should not always be 'an autistic style of interaction'. Whilst it is important not to insist that social is the only or best way, it is equally important to 'open up possibilities' for children to learn social meaning through social interaction (Nind, 2000). But social learning can be delivered via a teaching style that includes some aspects of an autistic learning environment. Essential to this approach is sensitivity to language use, understanding of the autistic perspective, provision of concrete experiences and, above all, the ever-present use of structure.

The importance of structure when using drama

I have found that what is critical for successful drama with children with autism is the use of a highly structured approach. A drama programme for autism should be properly planned and have some kind of developmental logic to it. It should unfold in a way that gradually builds skills, focusing on one thing at a time and pulling apart the smaller skill areas needed to develop a particular capacity. The fundamental issue of developing a child's capacity to perform pretend actions, for example, would need to be considered in terms of what it actually means 'to pretend' and the developmental steps that are involved in the achievement of this.

Approaches used with autism are very often prescriptive in nature, taking practitioners through clear stages of interaction or communication from which they are advised not to deviate (think of the Picture Exchange Communication System). The social-cognitive deficit that characterises autism means that ordinary assumptions about human behaviour and motivation do not apply. Prescriptive, highly structured approaches may feel restrictive to those using them, but have the benefit of limiting the possibility of acting on wrong assumptions. With this in mind, this book aims to provide activities that have clear and specific focus, that break down what the child needs to learn in relation to different capacities and that gradually build up skills.

By providing structure it is also possible to give an understanding of the autistic perspective, another element vital to good drama work with autism. Cumine *et al*, (1998) put it well by positing the idea of an 'autism lens' through which a better understanding of the perception and therefore experience of a person with autism can be gained. This book tries to provide some ideas about how to approach and teach certain aspects of drama to someone with autism, as well as address some autism-specific issues that regularly arise in group and drama work.

Developmentally informed work with children with autism

It is also important to take a developmental perspective in working with autism. To anyone who has worked in this area, it is apparent that children with autism can and do develop. As a teacher and therapist, I have known many children who, though lacking in most areas of social communication when young, have nevertheless gone on to develop skills in verbal communication, sociability, curiosity and playfulness.

Colwyn Trevarthan, in his authoritative text on children with autism, lists all the capacities that children can have in relation to the triad. For example, they may be able to form affectionate attachments, respond to others' emotions and have some skills for relating to the world. They can show communicative intent, understand symbols and be able to pretend, albeit in a rudimentary way (Trevarthan *et al*, 1996). Research has shown that though children with autism do deviate from the normal developmental path of ordinary children, the degree to which this is so varies greatly in each child (Cicchetti *et al*, 1994).

An important consideration is the diversity of the autistic population itself. It is clear that there are different levels of autism and that children vary greatly in their potential to progress. Evidence suggests the existence of neurological subgroups which have different combinations of whatever it is that causes autism and which mean that a child with autism can move through different categories of impairment (Leslie & Roth, 1993). Gillberg (2004) notes that a child diagnosed with classical autism who is speaking by the age of seven will probably go on to have Asperger Syndrome.

It is also probable that the causes of autism have a number of contributing factors. Some involve a primary biological disorder and some a secondary developmental delay, where what is impaired is closely related to the earliest capacities for social interaction, language, cognition and play. Indeed, work with autism often starts with the development of social relatedness in a child. Drama does contain the potential for engaging the individual and encouraging relatedness to others and to the world. Jennings (1995) has described how newborn babies come into the world as 'dramatic people', relating to others and to objects from the first hours of life.

This will be the starting point here, with Part I providing general ways of engaging the preverbal child using stimulus that is drama based and interaction that is dramatic in its content. Mirroring – the intentional copying of another person's actions and expressions – is a recurring theme in the book and will be used at different levels of ability, to engage and develop the child's capacity for reciprocal engagement. From facilitating communication through social engagement, the book will then move on in Part II to work that is programme based, to build specific skills using drama. The emphasis here is on group work, which is more facilitator led than child-focused. Areas of need that are commonly the focus of work with autism are explored in relation to a variety of drama techniques and games, and a range of activities provided.

PART I

Child-focused Work
Relating through drama

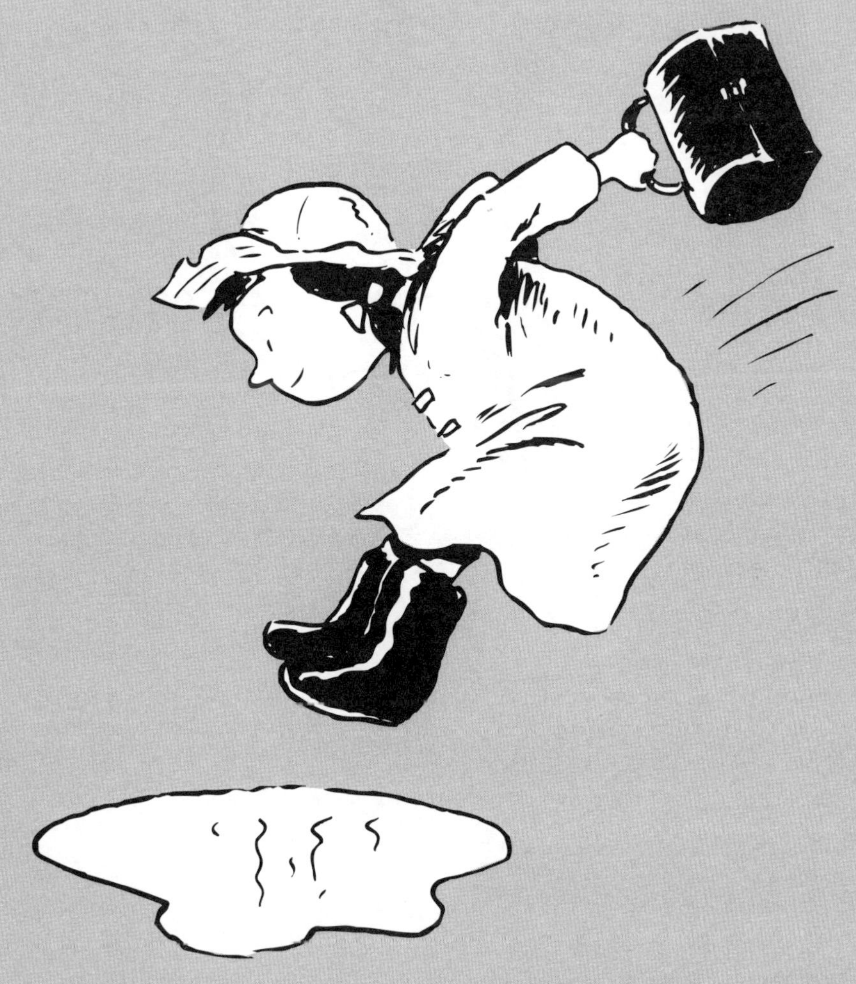

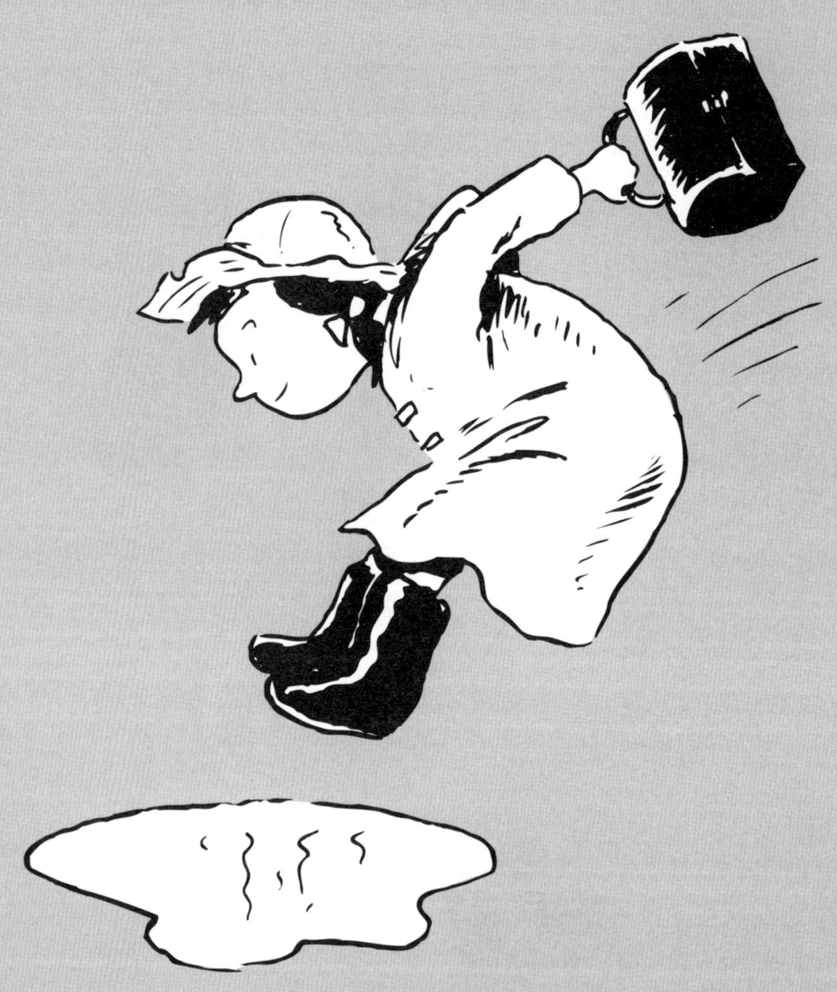

An Empty Space 1
Working with the sensory environment

Introduction

One approach to working with children with autism who are preverbal involves developing early skills in social interaction and play (Nind & Hewett, 1994; Christie & Prevezer, 1998; Hannah, 2001; Moor, 2002). Shared cooperation leads to cultural learning in all children. Skills in reciprocal social exchange and the sharing of a meaningful social 'space' underpin the later development of language and communication. Children with autism tend to avoid this kind of social contact, avoiding eye contact, withdrawing from cooperative play and being unable to share an interest in things with another person. A regular starting point for work with autism, therefore, is the simple engagement in acts of shared social meaning in relation to the world around or to another person.

This kind of work is often done through one-to-one interactions with the aim of facilitating communication and social relatedness through the sharing of mutually enjoyable activity. This interaction, moreover, usually uses sensory stimuli as a way of meeting a child where he is truly at. Children with autism operate in a sensory rather than social world, and using a non-social medium in interaction holds more potential in terms of real meaning (Williams, 1996). It is possible, for example, to follow the child's lead in sand play or play with water and encourage a little social sharing of a real though essentially sensory experience.

○ Sensory perceptual issues in autism

Since perception and sensory processing are primary difficulties in autism, it is where children are often 'at' in terms of their functioning (Gerland, 1996; Williams, 1996; Bogdashina, 2003). Donna Williams defines autism as difficulty in tolerating, processing and integrating sensory and perceptual information. She describes how the storing of information about an object, person or experience was for her based on the sensory or perceptual quality of that thing rather than any more generalised concept. As she writes, she knew a bowl by the inside of its shape, her word for it being 'whoodelly', derived from its sensory impact on her rather than any commonly known name (Williams, 1996). Williams points out that where sensory experience defines objects, it creates a language that cannot be easily shared.

○ Drama and sensory perceptual experience

At first glance, drama offers little in terms of sensory relating. It is the most socially oriented of the arts, involving actors, audience and a subject matter usually taken from life. Drama tends to concern the individual in relation to his environment, exploring what it means to be human in a social world. Peter Brook, in his book *The Empty Space* (1968), describes theatre as a 'small world' where life is presented albeit in a narrowed form. Nevertheless, Brook's ideas about theatre show how it might be possible to think about drama in ways that are sensory as well as social.

Brook makes the point that an important part of theatre involves the combining of life with art, the practical, aesthetic and often highly visual consideration of the colours and shapes of the set as well as the pitch and pace, intonation, rhythm and movement of the drama. In developing a performance, Brook describes how his first thoughts concern the subject matter together with the design so that, during rehearsal, he must always consider 'the height of the chair, the texture of the costume, the brightness of the light' (Brook, 1968).

Thinking of drama in terms of colour, light, texture, shape, movement and sound gives it potential as a sensory environment. Drama is said to involve a 'dramatic space' – Brook's 'empty space' – that can be filled in sentient ways to create a particular atmosphere or mood. Drama work with children with autism can focus on the making of an *environment*, one that promotes sensory experience but, by virtue of the fact it has been thought about, designed and made by people, gives a greater feel of human agency than that provided by a technology-based sensory room. Relating through one-to-one interaction can take place in and through this created environment.

The basis of interaction may be the sensory environment but, in the words of Margaret Donaldson, the 'human sense' of things in drama is never far away (Donaldson, 1978). Shared sensory experience easily slips into a more dramatic social way of relating, when that feels appropriate, through the introduction of social actions and routines suggested by the sensory stimuli. A sensory environment that involves a light switching off and on can prompt, for example, the social act of lying down and getting up and the language 'Good morning' and 'Good night'.

○ Interaction as a methodology

The methodology of interaction as an approach uses the ordinary model of learning in infancy (Christie & Wimpory, 1986; Nind & Hewett, 1994; Prevezer, 2000). This is characterised by regular social contact between an adult and child where the focus is the child and what he is doing rather than any designated outcome set by the adult. A key factor is the quality of the interaction itself, which should provide some sense of shared attention and pleasure, and thus of shared social meaning. Interaction should be slowed down and gentle with the aim of minimising the child's intolerance or fear of social approach and encouraging his accommodation to the adult and social learning per se.

O Features of early infant interaction

Typical of this experience in infancy is the creation of an emotional space between the parent or carer and the baby where a clear pattern of behaviour is established involving rhythmic, repetitive cycles of communication and reciprocity (Brazelton *et al*, 1974). In the early stages, it is the parent who mostly gains the baby's attention and who provides an overall frame for the subsequent interaction, but who does so with a good deal of sensitivity to the cues and affect level of the infant. Care is taken to respect the baby's need not to endure too high a level of excitement for too long a period of time.

In early interaction with an infant, the parent acts in a way that is especially lively, making full use of the voice, face, hands and smile and using expression that is often exaggerated or peculiar in some way. Daniel Stern (1974, 1985), writing about mother and baby-type interactions, found that the mother is highly attuned to her baby's activity and makes contingent responses, reflecting back that activity but in a way that is *not exactly mirroring*. Rather, she will pick out and amplify some action, expression or vocalisation of the infant, often attributing a meaning that is not necessarily clear. The mother relates in a way that is both familiar and understandable to the baby whilst moving the experience on just a little.

Similarly, the mother responds to the baby's activity in a way that reflects the intensity or quality of that experience as much as the actual content. Thus, she may respond 'cross-modally' where the degree of surprise or delight expressed in a baby's vocal expression 'Da!' is reflected back in the mother's raised eyebrows and open mouth of her facial expression. Stern argues that the baby experiences a range of sensations, perceptions, rhythms, actions and internal feeling states, but that it is through interaction and what is done there with these experiences that he begins to sort and cognitively organise them (Stern, 1985).

The findings of developmental psychologists such as Stern are reflected in more recent developments in psychobiology on how the mind works with the body and the importance of emotion to learning. What is becoming increasingly clear is that the development of cognition is not a separate process but is in fact strongly rooted in this process of organising social experience. Trevarthan (2006) points out that during early social encounters, focused attention in the body, which is characterised by some alignment of face, hands and body, together with the experience of emotion adds up to a thinking state. Facilitating social relatedness is thus about much more than enabling communication and promotes such capacities as a sense of agency, a sense of self, the ability to differentiate, to make connections and to 'think about' experience.

O Autism and interaction

The intuitive sociability and seeking out of engagement, witnessed in infants of only a few hours old, is rare in autism (Hobson, 2002). Children with autism show fewer of the behaviours typical of this kind of early interaction. They tend not to respond with anticipation to social invitation, do not often share an interest in something, and seldom imitate another person's actions or expressions. Any attempt to establish a cycle of communication usually breaks down rather than gains a rhythmic momentum. It is possible that autism means the absence of hardwiring in the brain that is the basis of these intuitive responses. It is also the case that problems with sensory perception and processing mean the individual may not be available for interaction in the first place.

When working through interaction, therefore, it is important to find the right balance between offering a small amount of stimulus whilst avoiding sensory overload. Gentle experiences of relating should both calm down the system of sensory processing and serve to 'move on' the child just a little. The aim is that the child should be able to tolerate stimulus and really take in the social experience offered. In this way, a greater capacity for social relatedness is gained and all that implies in terms of development.

O Assessment

An important preliminary to any work with interaction is an assessment of where the child is at in his functioning. Autism is a mixed bag in terms of the causes of behaviour and anxiety in an individual, and an assessment of a child's sensory perceptual functioning as well as of his level of attention and engagement is necessary. The Sensory Perceptual Profile in Olga Bogdashina's (2003) book, *Sensory Perceptual Issues in Autism and Asperger Syndrome*, is useful in gaining some understanding of what is going on for a child in terms of his perception and attention. The assessment profile in this unit will also help to establish a level for his ability to focus attention and engage in one-to-one interaction.

○ Session aims

Generally speaking, work that is child focused should aim to reduce the amount of stimuli present in the environment and slow down the whole pace of what is going on. Once stress levels and the likelihood of the child 'shutting down' are reduced, the development of the following capacities may then be more possible:

- interest in another person and what she brings
- willingness to explore the environment
- social responsiveness that is rhythmically organised
- intentional behaviour evident in the quality of anticipation and waiting
- cognitive behaviour evident in the quality of attention and aligned focus in the body
- enjoyment of social engagement.

○ The role of the facilitator

In order to achieve these aims, it is important for the adult working with the child to think and act in certain ways. She must:

- provide an environment that is predictable – through gentle, slowed down relating, sensitivity to the child's level of toleration and attunement to his affect. The child should lead, the adult taking their cues from the child's behaviour and activity rather than any desired outcome.

- provide contingent experiences – through mirroring responses that may also be cross-modal, exaggerated, out of the ordinary, or that mark out some aspect of the child's expression. In this way an experience that is safe and familiar whilst 'not exactly the same' is provided.

- promote the 'human sense' of interaction – by acting in lively ways with pleasure and a belief in the humanness of the child, attributing intention and agency in the child even where it is not clearly the case.

Unit 1   Assessment

Area of work: Focusing attention & sharing meaning in one-to-one interaction

Name of child:

Skills	Has this skill	Has demonstrated once with familiar adult	Demonstrates regularly with familiar adult	Demonstrates with another person
FOCUSING ATTENTION	✓	DATE	DATE	DATE
1 Allows adult to watch activity				
2 Accepts object handed by adult but puts to one side				
3 Accepts object handed by adult and incorporates into own activity				
4 Pauses in activity, synchronising actions with adult comments				
5 Briefly attends to an action performed by an object or adult				
6 Aligns hands, face or other parts of the body in response to an action or object				
7 Briefly follows a moving object				
SHARING MEANING				
8 Responds to an action or object with movement, gesture or vocal expression				
9 Remembers recent responses to an action or object				
10 Adopts adult's vocal expression, gesture or movement to accompany an action or use of an object				

Unit 1   Assessment *(Continued)*

Skills	Has this skill	Has demonstrated once with familiar adult	Demonstrates regularly with familiar adult	Demonstrates with another person
SHARING MEANING *(Continued)*	✓	DATE	DATE	DATE
11 Explores the environment outside of own personal space				
12 Explores objects other than favoured objects				
13 Sustains attention to an action or object				
14 Takes turns in an action or use of an object				
15 Anticipates what will happen with familiar actions and objects				
16 Looks from object to adult's face and back				
17 Is consistent in response to familiar actions and objects				
18 Shows pleasure in response to interaction				
19 Is consistent in different responses to different stimuli				
20 Takes part in social acts with objects				

Notes

____

____

____

____

____

Unit 1   Activities

<u>## Working with atmosphere and perspective</u>

The purpose of working with the environment is to encourage noticing behaviours in the child and the taking in of experience that is at once safe and knowable but also potentially rich in shared emotional meaning. The emphasis here is on sensory experience though there are elements of introducing a more social element if that feels appropriate. Working with the environment involves one or more of the following:

- creating an environment that has a particular atmosphere, for example, a particular quality of light or sound, or where the atmosphere can be switched from one thing to another
- setting up an experience where the environment is perceived in novel ways that are intriguing to the child
- working with objects that make a strong emotional impact by virtue of their shape, movement or noise.

1 Lairs

A lair is an enclosed space that is associated with the idea of shelter, hiding and careful watching. The visual artist, Louise Bourgeois, who made a concept piece entitled *Lair,* described it as a protective place to lie low and watch out for someone coming, a considered way of living for anxious people 'without strategy' (Bourgeois, 1998).

I have found that lairs can be very appealing to children with autism, who enjoy not only the getting in and out but also the being inside. Inside a lair, outside sounds are reduced and inside sounds are purer and simpler. Light is diffused and it is possible to create all sorts of lighting effects. You can build lairs that are dark inside, have low lighting, or lighting that can be switched on and off. It is also possible to work with sound by putting in objects that make a noise – a fan for example, or a ticking clock.

Lairs can be built of different types of materials and have different shapes, being long and thin, round, big or small. They can differ in terms of the interior atmosphere and have different ways of getting in and out. Tunnel entrances are often an exciting way to get in, as are a series of curtains. Children also love small doors and I sometimes build an alternative entrance/exit somewhere low down at the back of the lair. It is good to experiment to see what appeals most to a child and then recreate similar lairs over a period of time.

Daniel, aged eight, was hard to engage in any activity that was not of his choosing. He liked to play with things that poured – sand, water and rice – but would not allow anyone to join him in play, pushing away their hand or taking away their equipment. He appeared never to notice when a lair was being constructed in the corner of his classroom, yet, when it was ready, he would always go to the entrance without prompting. One afternoon, the teacher built a large, long lair with a blacked out tunnel entrance. Inside it was also dark though lit with some long travelling lights that were draped down the walls so that the light travelled downwards. A support worker waited in there too, with different gifts to greet the children as they arrived through the tunnel. For each child, she gave them something to eat and a glow-ball to hold. When it came to Daniel's turn, he received his gifts and then looked around the lair with interest. When he saw the curtain of moving lights, he pointed at it, looking back at the support worker and vocalising to get her attention. She looked with him and said, 'Lights, going dowwwn,' mimicking the movement of the lights with the sound of her voice. As she said the last word again, Daniel followed the movement of the lights with his gaze, moving it down in time with the word.

I like the idea of creating and dismantling different lairs, rather than building permanent ones. The repeated act of building a lair, creating each time one that is similar but cannot be exactly the same as the ones before, promotes this idea of mirroring a child's experience whilst moving it on slightly. Machines can replicate precisely but human beings cannot, and lairs are all about *human* creativity rather than technological intervention, though technology may certainly be used. Human agency is also present in the changing of the environmental atmosphere, when something is switched on or off, moved, turned up or dimmed. The fact that the lair is a pared down environment that can have one or two focus features unadulterated by other ordinary stimuli can give this sort of control much greater impact. Good building materials for lairs would be:

- parachutes of different colours (one dark, one light coloured)
- empty boxes
- tunnels
- fabric of different colours and textures
- curtains
- screens
- tents (particularly the supports to create a structure)
- hooks on the wall to hang material.

Good interior features of lairs are:

- lights (spotlights, glow lights, moving lights)
- cushions
- bedding
- low tables
- fans
- food and drink.

The essence of a lair is in its sensory and hidden features, and it is important to focus on the quality of the sensory environment you are creating. However, eventually you may want to introduce aspects of a more social world. For example, the interior of your lair may suggest a particular room of a house, the low-lit cosiness of a sitting room with a central glowing feature (television, fireplace), or the darkness-lightness-darkness of a bedroom, using a dimmer light and with bedding set out. I have found that even children who are quite solitary will join in with the act of lying down in darkness and getting up with light.

Another way of introducing the outside world is to add peepholes to the lair. Children can really enjoy being hidden and peeping out at the classroom world outside the lair or looking out for something that is passing round the outside of the lair, such as a toy, puppet or hand.

2 Perspectives

Some children can be intrigued by alternative ways of looking at the world and at people. Objects that give a different and novel viewpoint can be used to encourage a child to look and to relate. Looking down a tube, through a periscope or via a mirror can draw out a child, who may also be encouraged to look at people in this way. I have worked with children who would not look directly at someone, but enjoyed the experience of looking at my face through the end of a long tube. It is possible that this perspective reflects the child's own experience of people as disembodied body parts. It can certainly make children laugh.

Peepholes have already been mentioned in relation to lairs, but peepholes of all kinds can be effective. Doors with peepholes, looking into rooms through low peepholes and using boxes with peepholes that contain something inside can all be used.

3 Perception and emotion

There are certain objects the nature of which – their shape, movement, what they do – evoke powerful emotional reactions in all children. Examples of such objects would be:

- objects that disappear and reappear, such as pop-up toys or the open/close mechanism of a DVD player
- objects with holes through which things disappear for good, such as posting boxes and mouths
- objects that move erratically and may be noisy, such as Hoovers, jumping beans and jitter balls
- objects that flow, such as water, sand and glue
- objects with something sticking out, such as a button.

All children find such things fascinating and can react to them with a mixture of emotions, including wonder, anxiety, fear, excitement and joy. Children go through phases of finding one in particular fascinating, something about the object being emotionally meaningful to them in some way.

Children with autism can also be fascinated by such objects but in a way that is more isolated and less easily shared. Work can be done to help them share a little more the emotional impact of such an object. For example, other objects can be found that have the same features – shape, movement, noise – and therefore a similar emotional impact to the original object. Alternatively, the emotional quality of the favoured object can be expressed in another sensory modality, finding the right sound for the movement of the object – 'Da da!' for a pop-up toy – or translating the sound it makes into a movement.

4 Colour

There are many theories about the perceptual and emotional impact of colour, in art and religion, for example, as well as in education and therapy. We know that colour affects our mood and mental state, having the capacity to enliven us or calm and relax us. The importance of colour is, in fact, a vast subject that can be touched on only superficially.

What is important here is that, for some children with autism, the impact of colour on their inner state and sense of self can be significant (Williams, 1996). As a practitioner, I have noticed patterns of behaviour in children's response to different colours, particularly patterns in the level and quality of attention to certain colours. It seems to me that colour 'moves' children with autism in certain ways, specific colours evoking specific reactions.

⊙ snapshot *Sara*

Sara, aged five, went through a phase of using her Pixture Exchange Communication System to request a certain Lycra cloth in every session, taking off her shoes and lying on the floor in anticipation. Her key worker would fetch two such cloths of different colours and say, 'Choose'. Sara then lay on the cloth she had chosen and the key worker, together with another support worker, scooped up the edges and began to rock her in it.

Depending on the colour, there was a pattern to her behaviour once in the cloth. Inside the deep blue material, she would not make eye contact but rolled around in it as if she were a fish. Her movements were extraordinary and very beautiful, continually arching and curving her back and diving into the colour. In the red cloth, she was always alert, lying on her back and looking up at the two adults who held her with her eyes wide open, not moving much but interested in their faces. Inside the brightly coloured yellow cloth she tended to smile and laugh. The two workers sang her songs or talked to her in a way that seemed right for that colour.

Colour can be worked with environmentally, creating a 'colour world' which can be lived in for a while. The aim of drama work at this level is partially sensory integration but also an experience of 'being together' and relating in this particular colour. Coloured lighting may be suitable for doing this, but coloured cloth is really much better for getting inside a colour world. Cloth that is 100 per cent Lycra is especially useful, comes in a range of vibrant colours, is incredibly strong and allows children to be held in it, rocked and bounced.

It is possible to associate certain colours with the doing of certain activities, ones that are prompted by the emotional and mental associations of that colour. For example, blues and certain greens are meditative and good for activities that simply allow the child to be: to be held, rocked and sung to without requiring much in the way of reciprocity. Red is more arousing and can cause children to be more expressive with their faces. Face mirroring – copying the child's face expressions – or putting their expressions into sound – 'singing their face' – or working with a mirror can all be good ways of working in a red world. A nice bright yellow can bring out lots of joy and it is very good to be playful in yellow. It should be remembered, however, that response to colour is to some extent individual and you should first look to see what effect a colour has upon a child before deciding how to proceed.

Finally, it is good to work with the idea of being inside and outside of a colour as a way of marking the experience of the colour itself. This can be done by throwing the cloth in the air whilst holding on to the edges, then quickly dipping underneath so that you and the child meet inside the colour as it descends. Alternatively, you can set up different colour 'rooms', with appropriate activities and décor set out in each, and go from one to the other together.

5 Shape

The impact of shape is less well documented, yet it too can have a significant impact on the consciousness and emotional states of people with autism. Gunilla Gerland writes of her intense need, when she was a little girl, to touch objects that were curved. She describes how the experience of feeling a curve calmed her and gave her a sense of satisfaction: 'I kept touching things all the time – poking my fingers into or under bottles, sofa arms and door-handles, rubbing my palm against turned banisters...But no one around me had any idea it was the curve in particular that was the common denominator in everything I had to touch' (Gerland, 1996).

The pioneering German educator Friedrich Froebel believed that shape, like colour, has a language of its own, one that relates directly to nature and the visual world around and that impacts profoundly on our consciousness. He invented educational toys – his so-called 'gifts' – using building blocks, parquetry tiles, paper, modelling clay and sewing kits to promote play with two- and three-dimensional shapes that were round, square, linear and triangular. Froebel put forward the idea that shape holds meaning. The sphere, for example, with no flat planes, is an expression of motion and action, whilst the cube, with no curves, signifies inaction and rest (Brosterman, 1997). I find that round objects, such as balls, bring out an energy and liveliness in children and facilitate social acts between people (passing the ball). Similarly, objects such as beds, chairs and tables, used in play and in real life to perform less active behaviours, tend to have flat sides. When working with shape it is important to consider the forms found in an object. Does it contain:

- straight lines
- curves
- corners and edges
- gaps and holes
- protuberances
- patterns created by shape?

It is good to be exact about shape: how long or short are the straight lines, how big or small the curves, at what interval the gaps, and so on. It is then possible to work cross-modally, translating that experience into another sensory modality, trying to find a 'language' for the object to share and enrich the child's experience of its shape. Thus, the child can explore the object through sight or touch and the adult can provide 'the sound' of the object as he does so. Shape can be expressed in any of the following modalities:

- sound
- rhythm
- gesture
- movement.

Certain shapes prompt certain actions, and actions tend to give an engagement more social meaning. Objects with holes, for example, promote the act of looking through and possibly at someone. Round objects are good to throw and pass between you. Shapes that have corners and straight lines can be fitted together or made into longer and longer lines, and ones that are three-dimensional can be built into towers which can be sensationally knocked down. Shapes with buttons can be pressed, shapes with curves can be wrapped round something and objects with gaps can have things slotted in. All these actions suggest certain language – 'Gone!', 'Beep!', 'Ready, steady, go', 'Hello Sara!' – which adds to the social meaning. Though it is hard to anticipate what might appeal to a child, look out for things that are interesting or particularly tactile in terms of shape.

Working with opposites

One way of marking out a sensory or perceptual experience for a child is to move from it to its opposite and back again. Experiencing two opposite things, one after the other, has an extra emotional charge and more meaning in the sense that you know what it is in the light of what it is not. Working with opposites also satisfies the requirement in interaction that *peculiar* acts gain the most attention. Oppositional experience is always accompanied by vocal support from the adult, again as a way of marking it out and providing meaning. Examples of opposites would be:

- on–off
- light–dark
- in–out
- clockwise–anticlockwise
- hard–soft
- open–closed
- fast–slow
- rough–smooth
- up–down
- big–little
- loud–quiet
- warm–cold.

Choose play objects for their oppositional qualities, such as pop-up toys, toys with doors, flaps or lids, and similar toys of different sizes. You can also look for the oppositional elements within an ordinary object or activity. The possibility of switching lights on and off has been mentioned, but you can also work with high and low, up and down, fast and slow movements of an object, or the capacity of an object to be there and not there, seen and not seen. The tactile qualities of objects may be emphasised by choosing ones that provide opposing sensations or that can be one thing, full, and then another, empty.

Again, think in terms of the social actions suggested by the opposite. Open/closed gives rise to hellos and goodbyes, light/dark suggests 'Good morning' and 'Goodnight', fast/slow leads to getting tired and then getting ready to go again. Opposites can also lead to comments about feeling states; for example, 'rough/smooth' may prompt expressions of disgust and enjoyment. However, you need to exercise caution when working with opposites since the experience can be quite powerful and cause the child to feel overstimulated.

Mirrors

Imitation, the act of mirroring and of being mirrored, is crucial to the development of all children. Infants and their carers mirror each other from the first moments of life and go on to develop an increasingly sophisticated use of imitative behaviours. Children with autism can enjoy being mirrored too. For some, it may be the only interaction they will allow. The child's capacity in terms of mirroring can, in fact, be a useful way of assessing his general level of functioning and deciding on the best approach to use with him:

- Is a child able to notice that he is being mirrored?
- Does he enjoy mirroring-type interactions and seek them out?
- Is he able to mirror another person's actions himself?
- Is he able to mirror with confidence and creativity?

At its simplest level, with children who are hard to engage, mirroring may involve simply the use of an ordinary mirror. It is often the case that children with autism show great curiosity in a mirror, looking with interest, in the first instance, at themselves.

6 Looking in the mirror

When a child looks at himself in the mirror with curiosity then this should be the focus rather than any attempt at more social engagement. It is possible to provide a commentary whilst the child is doing this, to help 'point out' the child to himself. A helpful comment is, 'Here's Sam. Here's his head and here's his feet,' pointing out the full extent of the child. Children are often fascinated with themselves and will really look, but sometimes it is not clear that they know what they are looking at. As a child looks at parts of himself, his eyes, his mouth, his front, you can name the parts for him: 'Here's Sam's right eye. He's got two eyes. There's his left eye.'

⊙ **snapshot** *Saifur*

Saifur, aged ten, went through a phase of looking at himself in a small hand-held mirror. He particularly liked to look inside his mouth, tilting the mirror so that he could see what was in there. Setting his teeth in a clenched smile, he would look carefully at the front teeth, and then open wide to look along his back teeth. He looked at his tongue, waggling it in

It is good to be as specific as you can and to emphasise every so often that it is the *child's* body part you are describing, saying his name, to be clear about that too. It is also good to point out how one part of the body connects to another part, moving down from the head and pointing out how each limb is connected, as well as the hands and fingers and toes. At this stage, try to avoid references to your own body or self since this may confuse the issue.

7 Three-way mirrors

The child's fascination with himself can extend to fascination with what's inside. For some children with autism, dimensionality is an issue and they struggle to comprehend that the world is not made up of flat surfaces and of objects with no insides. Three-way mirrors can be used to point out to a child his own three-dimensionality, looking at him from the front, back and sides. It is also possible to get glimpses of parts of the body not easily seen with a plain mirror, such as the ears and how they are another way inside. As you point out parts of the child's body, you can ask them to move it: to move their shoulder blades up and down, tilt their head, or wiggle their bottom. The child may need help to do this but it does visibly demonstrate to him that this is indeed his body over which he has agency.

8 Looking in the mirror together

Eventually, a child might be ready to look at another person in the mirror. Communicating via a mirror is often more tolerable to a child with autism in fact, and may provide a first stage of relating (Rhode, 2001). The ordinary developmental pathway, from relating in a person-to-person way to relating to objects, often seems reversed in autism. The 'protoconversations' of early-type mother and baby interaction ordinarily precede an interest in objects (Trevarthan *et al*, 1996). However, in autism, the child may first relate to objects, with the adult observing or commenting but not directly intervening, and only later relate more directly in a person-to-person way.

The child's ability to tolerate looking at the adult in the mirror gives a good indication of what stage of relating he has reached. Is it possible to say, 'Here's Sam from head to toe. And here's Sally *(the adult)* too'? If it is possible, then a slightly different way of working is appropriate. Now it is helpful to differentiate between two people, pointing out the parts of the child and parts of the adult. You can say, 'There's Sam's hand and here's Sally's hand. Can they wave?' The use of the third person is helpful since it provides clarity.

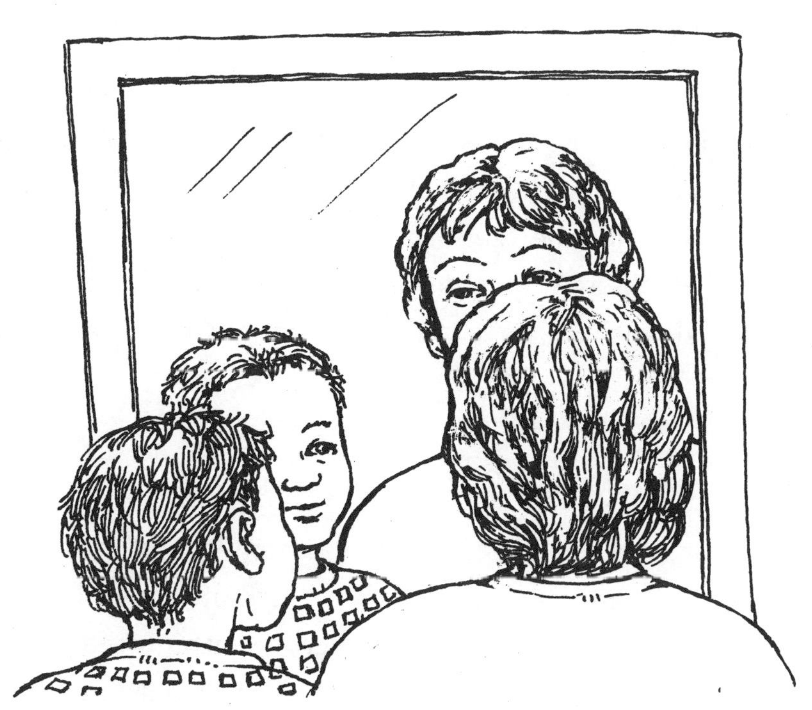

Things to do, say and look for

At this level of relating, it is often hard for the adult who is interacting with the child to know what to do and say. It is also hard to stay focused when the child himself feels mentally absent. However, staying focused and lively in interactions is vitally important and one aspect of the work. A child with autism may be relating to the world but in ways that are faint, indirect, delayed and easily missed (Alvarez, 1999). One way of working with this is to keep an observational state of mind: noticing, pointing out and trying to think about what the child is doing.

O Naming

You should use the child's name when referring to something he is doing or something about him, as well as the names of other people in the room. Be very clear about who is present and what they are doing. Naming can extend beyond people's names, however, to naming the part of the child's body that is doing something, naming the objects that he uses or the things in the room at which he is looking.

Describe what the child is doing, being specific about exactly what that is. I worked with a boy, Anthony, who would look through my different bags of toys but always avoided the bag of people toys. I tried to be specific about what he played with, 'You're playing with the car toys today', or 'Now you're playing with the animal toys'. After some months, when he did eventually start to use the people toys, it felt like a real development had occurred and something I could point out to him.

Naming feelings is more problematic at this level, but may be appropriate. In autism, a child has a disordered relation to his own body, and often poor awareness of self and how he feels. It is not always easy to know for sure how a child is feeling to be able to name it. However, putting a name to an inner feeling state can sometimes have a powerful effect on a child and can impact on his behaviour.

O Noticing and differentiating

Along with naming, noticing things about the child and differentiating clearly between one thing and another can contribute greatly to clarity and understanding in interactions. You can notice something that is different about the child, a new haircut or new shoes, or notice something that is the same, 'You've *still* got that cut on your finger'. Viola Brody (1997) plays with this idea of noticing when she suggests checking to see whether all the body parts of the child are still there. Are there still two ears, two arms, ten fingers and ten toes? You can also notice something about what the child is doing and differentiate between what he was doing just then and what he is doing now.

It is possible to differentiate one thing from another in the child's activity: 'You're passing me the *red* ball and now you're passing the *blue* ball.' Alternatively, you can say, 'That car is white with black stripes, that car is purple, that car has got a wheel that doesn't turn round properly.' You can differentiate between what the child is doing and what you are doing in response to that. Instead of saying, 'We're playing with cars', you can say, 'I'm giving you the cars and you're moving them around the room.' The relative nature of 'you' and 'me', however, means they are not that clear as reference points and the use of people's actual names is probably better.

O Making connections

Noticing, naming, describing and differentiating all help with the making of connections within experience for a child. It has already been discussed how being able to make connections between one thing and another contributes to the capacity to mentally organise, think about, understand and share experience. It may be the adult, persisting in a thinking and purposeful state of mind, who needs to see and point out these connections.

⊙ snapshot *Noah*

The teacher showed Noah, aged six, a spinner with the pattern of a wheel imprinted on it. She put a small yellow bag on to it that visually exaggerated the spinning action. Noah looked up from the small toy cars with which he was playing and watched. The teacher said, 'Round and round and round' in a rhythmic singsong way mimicking the action of the spinner. When the bag inevitably slipped off, Noah replaced it and waited for it to be spun again. He was enjoying this now, saying 'Again!' whenever the spinner stopped. However, after a few more turns, he picked up the little yellow bag and, holding it in one hand, turned back to his car toys. He seemed to have lost interest, the connection between him and the teacher gone. He took no more notice of the yellow bag though it remained in his hand. Eventually, the teacher pointed to it saying, 'Round and round and round' to remind him of what had just gone on, but Noah's face seemed blank and his eyes shifted up to the ceiling light. However, he did not 'lock on' to the light, as he had many times before, and

○ Marking change and endings

As with any approach to working with autism, it is important to note all changes to routine, to warn children that the end of the session is imminent and that holiday time is coming up. For a child with autism, social experience is hard to make sense of and organise in terms of time, and endings or changes can come as a shock. Use the child's visual timetable to provide information about the sessions. Incorporate symbol cards for the session itself, for when you are using a lair or working with a particular person, and note any change in time or day. Use a traffic lights system to begin and end sessions, where green is tapped to mark the beginning, amber to signify the near end, and red the end of the session.

Introduction

When we think about work with drama, we normally think of working with a group. Dramatic relating can occur on a one-to-one basis, but more often it takes place between a number of individuals. Drama reflects life, and most human life takes place in or relates to groups of people. Drama work with children can give a small taste of this, learning how to function in and negotiate interactions amongst people.

○ The purpose of a group with autism

For a child with autism, who is at the level of simply relating to people and the world, group work can be an effective way of working but needs to have a slightly different aim. It is less about giving the child an example of social relating that he can recognise and make sense of, and more an experience of the physical presence of other people. A group can provide a social environment that feels less intimate than one-to-one relating as well as one where other people can first be observed. From my experience of working with children with autism in school settings, I have noticed a clear pattern of development in those who are at this level, where beginning to notice other people and the world around, albeit in very swift glances, precedes actually interacting with those things.

Groups, moreover, have the effect of amplifying what is happening in terms of interaction. Virginia Axline, in her book on play therapy, writes: 'The addition of other children in the play contact brings out feelings and attitudes that could not show up in individual contact' (Axline, 1989). With autism, it may not be feelings that are brought out, but rather the sheer *presence* of others. A group of children performing some act together can wake up a child with autism to the fact that they are there and that something significant is going on.

Group ritual is important here since the routine of a familiar act, together with the repetition of each member of the group taking a turn to do that thing, can provide a very effective learning experience for a child with autism. Groups give rise to the clearest rituals since they allow something to be repeated most often. The numbers involved in a group also help to mark the fact that here is a discrete experience with a more definite beginning and ending than when two people come together.

○ Group structure

You should think creatively about who will be in the group. A group can consist of a number of children of the same age and ability, but it is possible to work with groups that are mixed. Some of the activities that follow, particularly those that involve some kind of imitative behaviour, may only be possible in a group with an equal number of autistic and non-autistic children. It is also imagined that there will be the support of at least one adult besides the group facilitator.

There are a number of ways of structuring a group. Using the model presented by Veronica Sherborne (1990) in her book on developmental movement, a group may be made up of partnerships of a child and an adult, or it can have a high ratio of adults who are providing support to children. Young children can be paired with older and more able children. There are schemes in operation in special schools where a partnership with the local mainstream schools involves a group of non-autistic children visiting regularly for a number of weeks to take part in a group and provide support. Many mainstream schools support inclusion and want to be involved in inclusive groups. Children, too, are often happy to be part of such a venture, see it as fun and can learn much themselves if their participation is properly valued.

Assessment of the needs of the group of children with whom you are proposing to work is important in informing your decision about how to constitute a group. Are the children generally at the level of only being related to? In this case a good deal of adult support will be needed. Are there signs of curiosity in others? Then less support will be necessary.

⊙ snapshot *Sophie*

Sophie, aged seven, attended a small class for children with Autism Spectrum Disorder in a resource base attached to a mainstream school. Though she avoided direct social interaction and had limited communication, she had begun to show an interest in other people and what they were doing, watching them from a distance. It was felt that small group work with an inclusive group of children would be of benefit to Sophie. Her teacher approached the mainstream school and asked if it was possible for a group of children to come to the resource base for a weekly 40-minute session. The school had a good inclusion policy and was involved in other integration projects. They were happy to be involved and a number of children were invited to join the group.

The teacher, with the support of one aide, facilitated the sessions. Work was done on noticing and mirroring others, and giving something to another person. Activities were fun and all the children enjoyed them. Both mainstream and resource base children took turns to be the focus of activities and the contribution of every child was valued.

The sessions made a strong impact on the visiting mainstream children. They would report back to their class teacher about each week's session, saying what they had done and what they had particularly enjoyed. Each week they looked forward to the next session and were disappointed when the group ended. Sophie and two of the children from the resource base who attended the group also enjoyed the sessions. After initially just watching and only taking part in activities with support, Sophie became more vocal and more spontaneous in her participation in activities.

The general aim of working with a group at this level is to encourage responsive behaviours, including awareness of others and what they are doing, and joining in with an activity. Work within the group will focus on beginnings and endings, as a way of encouraging awareness, as well as on providing simple activities that encourage a response in a child. It is important for the facilitator to be aware of the varying levels at which a child may respond within a group, from very swift glances at what is happening to enjoyment of activities and reciprocity of engagement. Aims should include the development of the following capacities:

- interest in other people and what they are doing
- sustaining interest, demonstrated by longer periods of looking
- ability to respond to greetings
- ability to recognise familiar activities and recall responses previously made
- coordination of personal activity/movement with that of the group
- following what others do in an activity
- enjoyment of group activity.

Unit 2   Assessment

Area of work: *Joining in with an activity*

Name of child:

Skills	Has this skill	Has demonstrated once in the group	Demonstrates regularly in the group	Has demonstrated outside the group
GREETINGS	✓	DATE	DATE	DATE
1 Notices hellos and goodbyes				
2 Can respond to hellos and goodbyes				
3 Notices when name is said or sung				
4 Enjoys greetings				
5 Can reciprocate a greeting phrase or gesture				
6 Recalls a greeting				
AWARENESS OF OTHERS				
7 Can pass on an object within a group				
8 Shows awareness of the presence of others in the group				
9 Shows interest in what others are doing				
10 Recalls an activity				
11 Coordinates movements/ sounds with others				
12 Takes cues from others in the group				

Unit 2 Assessment *(Continued)*

Skills	Has this skill	Has demonstrated once in the group	Demonstrates regularly in the group	Has demonstrated outside the group
AWARENESS OF OTHERS *(Continued)*	✓	DATE	DATE	DATE
13 Can wait for another when working in a pair				
14 Can coordinate movements with partner when working in a pair				
15 Can cooperate with partner when working in a pair				
16 Enjoys group activity				
17 Enjoys being chased				
18 Can chase others				
19 Can notice the whereabouts of others in a game				
20 Will look for others who are hiding				

Notes

____

____

____

____

____

____

____

Unit 2 Activities

Beginning and ending rituals

A ritual is an act performed regularly, usually at a designated point in the proceedings of a group. Rituals may be very ordinary acts, such as saying hello or sharing a snack, which become ritualistic by virtue of the fact that they are repeated on a regular basis, carried out intentionally and with meaning. Indeed, it is in the familiarity and repetition of the act that the power of the ritual is held. Children, including those with autism, often anticipate, participate in and really enjoy a ritual, appreciating the familiarity of the act. Efficacy is an issue here, since children often gain satisfaction from knowing what is expected and how to respond.

1 Hello songs

Children often respond better to being sung to rather than talked to. Anything can be said in a 'hello' song since it is really an opening conversation addressed to the child in a singsong way.

Instruction

1 A 'hello' song may simply involve singing 'Hello' to the children in the group, naming each in turn: 'Hello Jack, how are you?'
2 You may or may not require a response from the child, depending on his ability.
3 You should say hello to all members of the group, including other adults or helpers present.

Variation

Alternatively, a 'hello' song may be a familiar song, particularly one favoured by the children, which is sung at the beginning of each group. With older and more able children, I sometimes use a repertoire of three or four songs and ask them to choose which we will sing that day.

2 Musical names

Another way of saying hello to children and pointing out their presence in the group is to find an individual rhythm for each child's name.

You need

A variety of instruments, one for each member of the group.

Instruction

1   Choose an instrument for each child. Choose one that will match the sound and number of beats in the name.
2   Instruments can also be matched to the personality of the child.
3   Sitting in a group, say hello to the child, saying their name and using the instrument.
4   Repeat this a few times and at the beginning of each group.

3 Rolling the ball

The liveliness of a ball rolling across the floor creates a social connection that is also quite gentle.

You need

A special ball, the same ball used each week.

Instruction

1   Begin the group each week by sitting on the floor and rolling the ball to individual children, saying hello as you do so.
2   Encourage the children to roll it back, offering them support if necessary. However, it often pays to wait so allowing a little time for the children to roll the ball back by themselves.

4 Move and touch

This is an activity for more able children and is a good way of saying hello to the space and to each other.

Instruction

1   Begin groups by telling the children to go and touch different parts of the room: 'Touch the door', 'Touch the window'.
2   Change this to different parts of people: 'Touch Mona's leg'.

5 Goodbye songs

As with 'hello' songs, a 'goodbye' song can simply be singing goodbye to each child in turn.

Instruction

1   Use a special 'goodbye' tune to sing: 'Goodbye Helen. See you next week.'
2   Go round the group, singing to each child in turn.

Variation

You can also use a set song which you sing at the end of the group, though you should always say goodbye to each child as well, naming them.

6 Blow out the candle

Children are often drawn by the liveliness of the flame and quickly understand what is expected of them in this activity.

You need

A thick candle that can be used for many weeks and which will provide continuity to the ritual. An automatic lighter.

Instruction

1 With the children sitting in a circle, so that everyone can be seen, take the candle on a holder round to each child.
2 Sing goodbye to the child and encourage him to coordinate the blowing out of the flame with the ending of the song.

Comment

The ritual really works best in a space you can darken.

7 Gifts

The act of opening and receiving something can be meaningful even to a child who is quite withdrawn.

You need

A special box with a lid and items to go in the box such as: small sweets, pieces of fruit, the children's names on individual labels, small interesting objects such as feathers, flowers or ribbons.

Instruction

1 Pass the box round the group, with each child encouraged to choose one thing from it as a gift.
2 The child then passes the box to his neighbour until everyone has a gift.

Variation

You can provide a 'Pass the parcel' package from which children remove a sheet to find something for themselves.

Whole group activities

It is helpful to have an element of support in the groups that follow: adult helpers or the support of more able children. The degree of support necessary depends on the ability of the children involved, but the participation of helpers in an activity, taking turns with the children, usually improves the pace and overall success of the group.

8 Put your feet in the centre

I have worked with a number of children with autism who prefer communicating through their feet than with their faces and who really enjoy this type of activity.

Instruction

1 Tell the children to take off their socks and shoes.
2 Sitting in a circle, encourage the children to move into the centre so that all your feet are meeting.
3 Wiggle your toes as if they are saying hello to each other.
4 Name whose feet are whose and say hello to individual toes.
5 Encourage pairs of children or child and adult to push away from each other with their feet and return to the edge of the circle.

9 Pass it on

Some children who at first find this activity difficult and need support for it are often eventually able to join in independently.

Instruction

1 The leader starts the activity by touching a body part of her neighbour, making a sound as she does so: beeping the nose, buzzing the knee, creaking as you pull on the ear.
2 Encourage the neighbour to pass this on, beeping the nose or whatever to his neighbour on the other side.
3 You may initially need to help with this, perhaps doing the action yourself at first, but children usually learn to do it themselves eventually.

Comment

Some children with autism are hypersensitive and find it hard to be touched. Others love work that involves touch, seeking it out at every opportunity. You need to assess the tolerance of the children with whom you work and decide how much touch, if any, is appropriate.

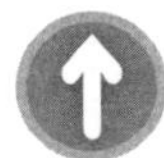

10 Group cradling

In a small group, take turns to rock children in the Lycra cloth.

You need

A large sheet of Lycra cloth.

Instruction

1 Ask for a volunteer or select one child. Ask him to remove his shoes.
2 Have the child lie down on the cloth on his back.
3 Encourage the other children to hold the cloth and help with the rocking.
4 Ensure that no one puts their leg in the way of the cloth since this will then bump the child who is being rocked.
5 Ensure each child has a turn in the cloth.

11 Camping

You need

A large sheet of dark-coloured cloth or a parachute, and a light.

Instruction

1 Sit in a circle with the cloth or parachute spread out in the middle and the light, if you are using one, underneath that, next to an adult who can look after it and switch it on.
2 Take a little time to say hello to the group and then encourage everyone to hold on to the cloth and get ready.
3 Tell them that they should pull the cloth up and over their heads so that the whole group will be sitting inside it. You may need to do it a few times just to give children the idea of what you are trying to do.
4 When you are inside the cloth, switch on the light and greet everyone again.

Comment

The effect of the whole group going under the cloth at the same time is a dramatic change in atmosphere. Dark cloths work best since they provide the greatest transformation in light. Once inside, switching on a light changes the atmosphere again, into something more cosy and genial, and children usually love this. Getting the cloth over everyone's head at the same time, however, is quite a skill and often needs some support workers, placed at regular intervals around the circle, to achieve.

12 Group mirroring

This is the least intimate of the many mirroring activities that are described in this book. It is also the simplest since it requires only the child who is the focus of the activity to be copied.

Instruction

1 Tell the group that they are going to copy one child. The child himself may not take in at this point that he is the focus, the aim of the activity being that he will eventually realise this.
2 Sit in a circle in the manner of the child who is the focus.
3 Copy the movements that he makes, encouraging the other children to do the same.
4 Do this for a little time, keeping careful note of the focus child's level of awareness, the extent to which he will wait for others and his general enjoyment of the activity.
5 Allow other children a turn to be copied so that no one feels left out.

Comment

This activity only works if there is a sizeable proportion of quite able children in the group, who are prepared to copy another and who can do it with some skill. For the child who is the focus, once he notices what is happening, the experience can be highly enjoyable. I have known children who will start to move with deliberation, waiting when necessary for the group to catch up with them, and who can carry on the activity for some time.

13 Photo album

Many children with autism, who are withdrawn, relate more readily to photographs of people than to real-life people, and it is often a good idea to make a photo album of the children when a group begins to meet.

You need

A camera, some labels and a scrapbook.

Instruction

1 Take photographs of all the group members, children and adults.
2 Compile an album of photos and names, one per page.
3 Use the album to support some of the group's activity. For example, greetings can incorporate a photograph, 'Here's Courtney' (looking at her photograph). 'Is she here today?' (looking for her). 'There she is! Hello Courtney.'

Comment

Talking to someone via a photograph slows down the interaction, giving the child a little more time to process what is being said and that it is being said to them. I find that a photo album of the group, which children look through at leisure, also helps with the learning of who is actually present and what their names are.

You need to consider carefully who is partnered with whom. You can choose from the following options: child-child, child-older child, autistic child-non-autistic child, child-adult. It is often best to carry out a paired activity with the rest of the group looking on. In this way, you can provide a good deal of support to the pair who are working together whilst the other children have an opportunity to watch, which is in itself a valuable exercise.

14 Pairs

Lots of fun can be had with this playful activity.

Instruction

1   Put the children into pairs.
2   The leader calls out different body parts – feet, hips, backs, noses, and so on – and the children must match those parts of their body together.
3   Pairs wait for the next body part to be called.

Comment

Very often, children who do not quite understand the activity at the outset quickly learn what is expected and have fun with it. Be aware, however, of children who do not respond well when touched since this is essentially a touch exercise.

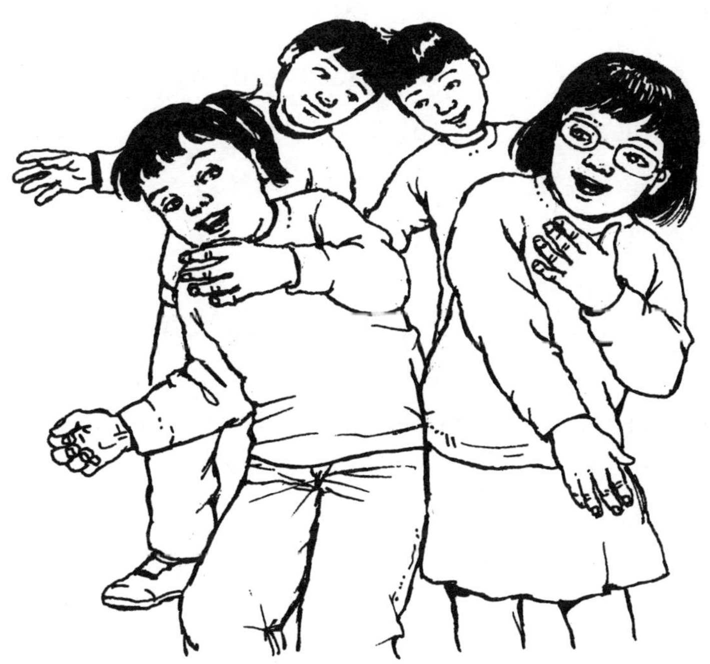

15 Trust lead

This activity builds a sense of trust between two children.

You need

Items for an obstacle course including, tables, chairs, tunnels, ramps, bollards.

Instruction

1 Clear a space in the room and set out an obstacle course.
2 Add interesting elements to the course, such as things that are crawled through, stepped over and walked between, but do ensure that the course is safe.
3 In pairs, group members take turns to lead their partner through the course.

Comment

A child may both lead and be led by their partner, or may just have one of these roles, depending on what he is able to do.

Variation

The activity can be carried out in a variety of different ways:
◎ with or without blindfolding the child who is being led
◎ leading by holding hands or leading by the partner making sounds.

16 Coordinated movement

This activity is typical of the cooperative movement work of Veronica Sherborne. More ideas for similar activities can be found in her book, *Developmental Movement for Children* (1990).

Instruction

1 Provide an activity where partners must coordinate their movements. This may involve one jumping on a trampoline and the other holding his hand, one helping the other to balance whilst walking along a beam, or one riding on the back of another as if riding a horse.
2 Encourage partners to take turns in the chosen activity.

Good group games

Children who are just beginning to relate to others love to play chasing games. Games that are successful with such children usually involve some kind of chasing, with the child being chased rather than chasing another. When we are imitated by others our heartbeat goes down, but when we imitate it goes up, so being chased is a less stimulating and overwhelming experience, though exciting enough for a child with autism.

With games of chase, you must consider how you will organise them since they do require adults or more able children and children without autism who are prepared to chase.

17 Duck, duck, goose

Instruction

1 Sit in a circle, on the floor or on chairs.
2 Select one child and instruct him to walk around the outside of the circle.
3 As he walks, he touches each group member on the head saying, 'Duck, duck, duck'.
4 When he touches one person he says, 'Goose!'
5 That person then jumps up and chases him around the outside of the circle.
6 The first person tries to sit down in the now empty space before the 'goose' can tag him.
7 If he does so, the 'goose' becomes the person who calls out 'Duck, duck, goose'.

18 Stuck in the mud

Instruction

1 One person is 'it' and holds out his hands with the fingers spread, and all the other children hold on to a finger.
2 Agree on a word as the signal to run. This may simply be 'One' or 'Blast off!' when counting down from ten, or it may be 'Go' of 'Ready, steady, go'. For children who are more able, the signal can be any ordinary word put into a short story or list of things, such as 'banana' in a list of fruit.
3 The first child starts to speak, using the signal at some point, at which the other children run away.
4 The child who is 'it' chases and tries to tag them.

Sometimes children are able to play games that do not involve chasing, but may first need coaching in how to play. 'Hide and seek' is a good example of this. I find that children with autism have great difficulty with this game, particularly the idea that, when they cover their eyes, children hide but are still 'there' in some way. In fact, the game has all kinds of implications in terms of developmental competency and requires an understanding that things which are not visible can still be present. A child's ability to play the game often indicates his developmental level in terms of object permanence and theory of mind. However, some children can learn to play the game as part of a general programme of developing skills and understanding. In any case, as children develop in other ways, their capacity to play such games as 'Hide and seek' invariably develops as well.

The next two games are simple versions of hiding games and serve as precursors to 'Hide and seek'.

 19 Jumping Jacks

Instruction

1   One child is 'it' and stands facing a wall. The other children line up a short distance away, facing him.
2   The children move forwards in bunny jumps.
3   The child at the wall turns to look at the others, every so often or after the count of 'five', to see if anyone is jumping.
4   He points at any child who is jumping, who should then stop.
5   The first person to jump to the wall becomes 'it'.

20 Hide and seek in the open

Instruction

1   Establish the number of children who are playing the game.
2   One child is 'it' and counts to ten covering his eyes.
3   The other children scatter, stopping when ten is reached.
4   The child who is 'it' uncovers his eyes and points to all the children he can see, counting them out.

PART II

Group Work
Building skills

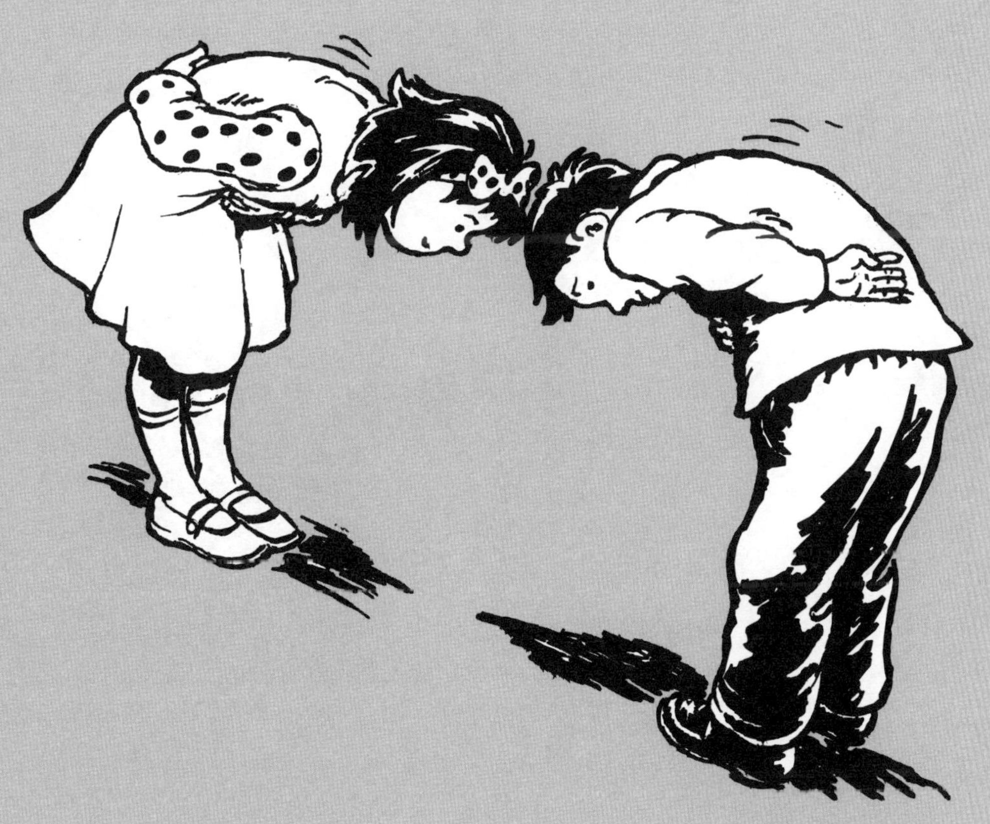

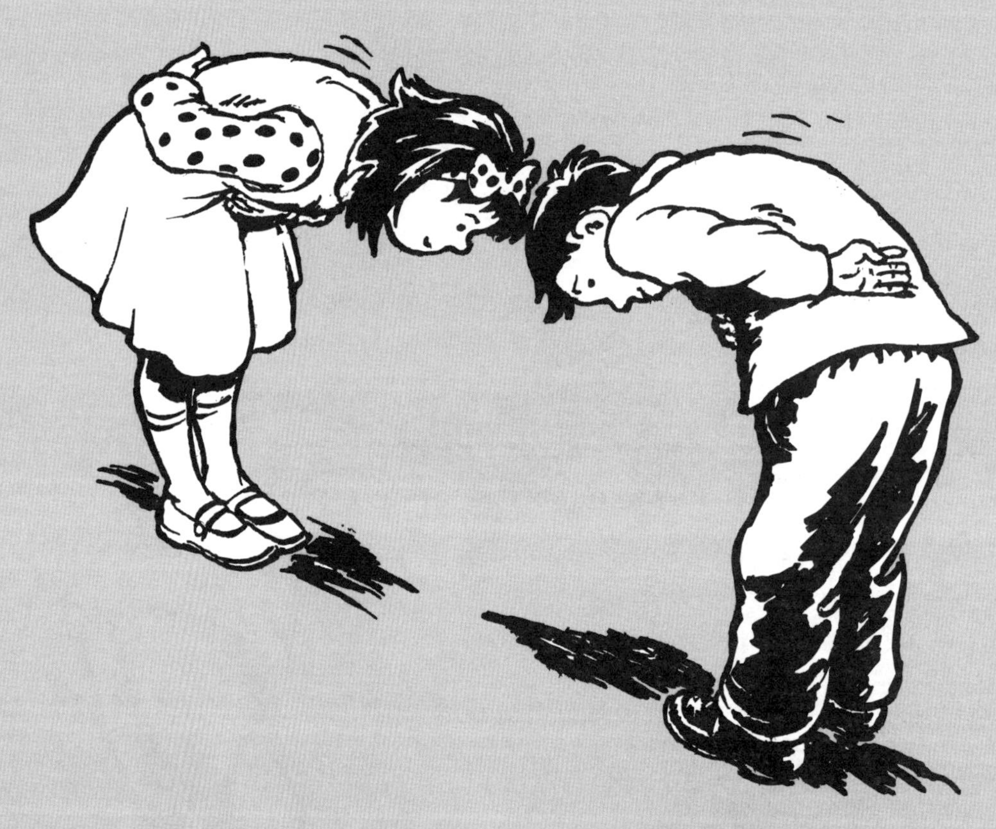

In Part II the focus of the work shifts from following the child's lead to working in a way that is more group oriented and facilitator led. The emphasis here is on delivering a programme of work aimed at developing specific skills using drama techniques. Drama offers a wonderful opportunity to develop understanding and practise skills in social communication and works well in developing physical and vocal expression, the ability to pretend, to role play, to make narratives and to think creatively. However, drama work needs to be carefully structured so that the child with autism is able to take part and really contribute.

Putting together a group

Most of the activities outlined in the following units are designed for small groups. Group size can vary, between, say, three and ten, depending on the needs of the child in question and the nature of the activity itself. Some activities need a larger group to really be effective and some work well with just a few children. Where a large group of children is necessary, of at least eight, the activity is marked 8+ .

In putting together a group, it is important to remember that it should not be a 'special needs group' per se. Whilst it is recognised that children with autism often make friends and want to interact with other children who are on the spectrum, the premise here is that they should also have the opportunity to interact with and learn from non-autistic children who can provide good models of interaction, communication, expression and creativity.

Groups may consist of only one child who has autism or of a few children with autism, but a number of children without autism will usually be involved too. Increasingly, children with autism are being included in ordinary schools, and a part of the work is about enabling non-autistic children to respond more effectively to their classmates. An inclusive group that is successful is one where children are equally valued and properly heard, however, and all children should have a turn at being the focus of an activity.

Group techniques

There are a number of techniques, commonly used in group work with children, which are referred to in Part II:

○ Circle time

Many of the activities in Part II involve the group sitting in a circle, or at least beginning in a circle. In primary education, 'circle time' is well established as an approach to enhancing children's interpersonal skills. Children sit in a circle, on chairs or on the floor, so that everyone can see everyone else. Staff, including the teacher, are a part of the group, and the main method of working is through speaking and listening, with little work done on paper. Circle time is highly adaptive, allowing work to be done that is different in aim and content, but carried out using similar methods. A circle should also be an 'emotionally safe place' where people learn how to listen, respect others and express how they feel (Mosley, 1998).

Autism education in mainstream education popularly uses a circle time approach, known as 'Circle of Friends', to help include a child with autism in the peer group. Circle of Friends is a peer support system which uses the collective strengths of a group of peers for the benefit of a 'focus individual', though participation in the circle should ultimately be beneficial to all group members. The idea is that a selected group of able children should problem solve issues of friendship and social interaction and offer strategies to the student in question, providing both practical and emotional support and helping to bring about changes in behaviour (Taylor, 1997).

As an approach, Circle of Friends has a particularly satisfying quality, offering a way of working that is at once supportive, gentle, creative and highly relevant socially. The method is adapted here in that the group are asked to 'think for' the child with autism, if that is necessary, providing him with the creative ideas needed for drama.

○ Brainstorming

Brainstorming is another method of generating ideas within circles. It generates ideas quickly, abundantly and in a way that involves the whole group. Done properly, brainstorming has the added effect of building positive group feeling since all contributions are welcomed and accepted without validation.

Brainstorming involves the teacher asking the group to think of as many ideas as they can on a given subject. She then writes down all contributions, adding ideas of her own if she wishes. There are a few important things to remember when brainstorming:

- accept all contributions without judgement
- do not rank contributions in any way, but give each equal value
- allow pauses to occur and wait patiently for more ideas to come
- allow the brainstorm to come to a natural end.

In Part II, the use of brainstorming is suggested where activities require a number of ideas on one topic, for example, when writing scripts for everyday situations.

Modelling and partnering

For a child with autism placed in a school setting, a typical developmental pattern is an increasing curiosity in other children, shown initially in brief, almost imperceptible glances and later on in really looking. Looking at others, at what they do, how they do things and imitating them, is an important element in the development of all children and is partly how children learn.

Modelling is a group technique that promotes the idea of looking at someone doing something. For example, you ask one child or a small group of children to show something to the rest of the group. All other group activity stops and everyone's attention is drawn to what is being modelled. In drama terms, this would be a prototype actor and audience situation, though what is being modelled may be very short and simple indeed.

For the child who is the focus of the group, modelling can be used developmentally so that he is first provided with the opportunity to watch only, and later invited to model himself or be part of a group. Be cautious about forcing too much eye contact and allow the child to look in his own way and in his own time. Partnering can also be used to give the child in question the opportunity to work with and 'take in' the experience of another child, though partners often need to be carefully selected.

Leading and following

Finally, it is important to consider activities in terms of who goes first and who second. In the early stages of group work, it is probable that the child with autism will not follow the lead of others, and can only be followed, his movements or sounds copied by other children but not reciprocally. It is necessary to work with this and encourage the other group members to do the same. This is why more mature children often need to be in the group, since young or immature children find it hard to follow others themselves. In following the child who is the focus of the group, other children can be encouraged to be more responsive to what that child does, learning how to prompt and knowing when to give more time.

Generally speaking, the instructions in the activities section assume the group facilitator is the leader, but it is a good idea to vary the leader role, allowing children to take a turn to lead.

Structure of the session

Drama sessions which have a set format help to establish a sense of predictability and safety. In particular, attention should be paid to such things as routines and rituals, repeating familiar activities and thoroughly practising the skills that are being taught. In Part II, the activities become progressively more complex and challenging, but all the sessions should generally go through the following steps:

- Greeting
- Warm-up
- Developing trust
- Focus skill
- Ending.

○ Greeting

A group session should begin with some kind of opening ritual: either going around the circle to say 'hello' to individual members, singing a 'hello' song or, for older children, greeting the group and saying how they feel that day or something they have recently done.

○ Warm-up

Design warm-up activities to encourage the individual to focus on himself, the other people in the group and the room. They can also warm up the body, voice or imagination, whichever is needed for the main activity that is to follow. Warm-ups may involve listening to sounds outside the room, in the room and within yourself, or relaxing and listening to a piece of music or guided visualisation. Suggestions for warm-ups are included here with the main activities.

○ Developing trust

In a sense, the way that the group is run should establish a degree of trust between the group members, so specific activities may not be necessary. Many of the exercises and games given in the following units will incidentally build

 USING DRAMA WITH CHILDREN ON THE AUTISM SPECTRUM

trust and group cooperation. Activities such as mirroring, leading someone who is blindfolded, sharing information about yourself and being the focus of an activity all help to build trust. However, it is often the case that the child with autism is perceived by others as an outsider and this means activities to 'gel' the group are particularly important. This is especially the case for older and more able children with autism who have greater self-awareness and therefore awareness of their 'difference' from the other children.

○ Focus skill

Before planning a programme of work, an assessment of where the child is at in terms of dramatic ability is needed. Depending on which area of dramatic skill you decide to focus, activities can be selected from the relevant part of the book.

⊙ example 1

Andrew was assessed as having a small amount of skill in symbolic play: moving a car along the floor and making driving noises, taking it to the garage to fill up with petrol. It was felt that work was needed to develop his ability to pretend. He was assessed using the profile in Unit 3 on developing pretence and physical expression. It was found that, though he could 'independently transform one object into another of similar shape', he could not mime an action without the support of a prop. Activities were used from the section on 'Pretend actions' with some more work on using imaginary objects to increase his skill here.

⊙ example 2

Nicky could recognise a range of emotions, beyond the basic four, in pictures of faces. She could also give a realistic reason for why a character in the depiction of a scene was displaying a particular emotion. However, she could not say any more than this and often got frustrated when certain incidents happened to her. She was assessed using the profile from Unit 6 on awareness of self and others. This showed that, though she had a basic understanding of emotion, she was unable to discuss such things as the intensity and quality of a feeling. Activities from the section on feelings were selected, particularly those that related to identifying and thinking about the feelings involved in recent situations. When further work was carried out using activities to explore the intensity and quality of feelings, Nicky was more able to contribute.

Jim had ability in terms of language, play and general social skills. He could respond in conversation and was able to discuss social incidents and stories. However, he was not very good at reading other people's body language to gauge how they were feeling. His responses in everyday social situations were often not quite right and were off-putting to other children. Consequently, he tended to be isolated in terms of his friendships.

It was felt that Jim could learn more about everyday interactions through the use of improvised drama. He was assessed using the profile in Unit 8 on improvisation and it was found that he was weak in terms of his capacity for reflection in drama. He was generally unable to make comments about a character's motivation or possible reaction. Work was done with Jim using the drama technique of Playback, where Jim could watch and rehearse dramatic situations that were based on his ordinary everyday social interactions.

Please be aware that some activities form part of a developmental sequence and should follow the order set out in the book. It is worth thinking about repeating activities since repetition and routine are such important parts of work with autism.

O Ending

Just as there is an opening ritual to each group, so there should be some kind of closing ritual. This may be a 'goodbye' song or simply a plenary of what has taken place in that session. Making a good ending to a session is a crucial part of the work for two reasons. First, knowing when something has come to an end is always important for someone with autism. Second, where dramatic play has taken place, it is important for children to 'de-role' from whatever imaginary activity they have carried, to come back to being themselves and be ready to return to class. For more on endings see Unit 9.

The role of the facilitator

The teacher or group facilitator needs to keep in mind the following points:

- a clear structure – to ensure access to learning for the child who is the focus of the work, always think in terms of structured drama. Unless a child is very capable, try not to leave activities too open. Teach one thing at a time, considering carefully what it is you are actually asking the child to do.

- safety – ensure that the creative space you are offering feels safe. This is achieved through the predictability of repetition and routine, the provision of structure, as well as the gradual development of group trust.

- playfulness – children with autism are children and quite often love to have fun, play games and participate in enjoyable activities. It is lovely to see a child develop in his capacity to be playful, to tease and joke and enjoy himself with others.

- reciprocity – in working with autism, one of the most important resources available to you is the responsiveness of other children. Use the sessions as an opportunity to develop this, providing activities that allow the children to really interact, rather than simply share the same physical space, as is so often the case. Find a way of being together that is meaningful to and enjoyed by all.

All in all, the role of the facilitator is to strike the right balance between providing a learning environment that is sufficiently structured and thought out to ensure full participation, whilst giving space for creativity and expression and allowing the child with autism to 'simply be'.

3 Sculpting
Using the body/starting to pretend

Introduction

Focusing on the body, developing awareness of its different parts and ability to express meaning physically, is an important area of work in autism. Drama is a body-based art form, where the actor conveys ideas, relationships and emotion through his face, hands, movement and voice. Given the importance of the body, there are any number of techniques in drama to develop body awareness and its use.

Sculpting is one such technique involving the adoption of a physical position to show an action, feeling or relationship. The adopted pose must convey something that may be based in reality but is essentially imagined. Examples of sculpts would be: the physical act of pushing something, conveying through body language the feeling of anger, the relationship between a mother and child. Individuals can create their own sculpts by freezing their body position and facial expression, or they can be moulded by another person. The effect is of a statue which can be appreciated by others, walked around, viewed from different angles and brought to life. It is possible to make group sculpts, where people are positioned in relation to each other, to create a scene or 'tableau'.

In its use of stopping and reflecting, the pace of work with sculpting is quite slow. Sculpting focuses on the body – posture, gesture and facial expression – and is explicitly concerned with the *outward* appearance of things, though it may attempt to convey an inner state. It is related to mime in that it is not concerned with verbal expression, but differs in the way that it allows experimentation and practice of different positions.

○ Autism and pretence

Sculpting is a form of *representation* – the imagined reproduction of a real experience – and requires the person to pretend. Pretence is, of course, something with which children with autism have difficulty. Autism involves an impairment in imaginative thought, in the forming and manipulating of mental images of real experiences, so that a child with autism has a deficit of socially meaningful mental material upon which to base a pretence. Many children with autism also have motor coordination difficulties which impact on body awareness and control, and the ability to perform any action, pretend or real.

Some of the activities offered here will involve building the capacity to pretend in simple and gradual stages, developing both the body and the imagination. To do this, it is helpful to consider what actually happens when someone 'pretends', in particular, to look at how children develop their ability to carry out pretend play.

○ What is pretend play?

From birth, children move through different stages of playful engagement with the world, from interactions with their carer, to exploration and manipulation of objects, to more and more complex combinations of the two. Figure 3.1 on page 54 gives an outline of the basic stages in the development of a child's capacity for play.

It is important to remember that the different human capacities for cognition, sociability, language and play do not develop in isolation, but are closely connected, building one upon another from the earliest stage. The development of language and symbolic play, for example, is related so that a child who exhibits higher language abilities will also have more mature symbolic play. Moreover, the later development of representational capacities, such as language and symbolic play, comes out of earlier skills in non-verbal interaction. The ability to symbolise requires skills in sharing joint attention, joint referencing, processing social experiences, and imitation – that is, all the capacities acquired through early non-verbal experiences of social interaction between a baby and its carer (Cicchetti *et al*, 1994; Trevarthen *et al*, 1996).

Children without special needs begin to show the capacity to perform pretend actions with real objects from the age of nine months and go on to develop increasingly sophisticated pretend behaviours. In the early stages, pretend actions are almost identical to real actions so that pretence is closely related to memory, what Piaget (1954) described as 'deferred imitation'. The development of pretence (see Figure 3.2, page 55) depends on the ability to 'decouple' experience, in all its social, emotional and cultural richness, from current real-life perception, and to hold it as a mental image that can be retrieved and manipulated (Leslie, 1987).

One-to-one interaction *(0–6 months)*
Direct face-to-face relating
Imitation, rhythm and turn taking
Play with body parts
Joint attention
Awareness of presence and absence

Manipulative/Exploratory *(6 months)*
Reaching for and exploring objects
Sensory experience of object

Relational/Organising *(9 months)*
Sorting and combining objects
Putting in/taking out
Putting two things together
Cooperative awareness
Relating via objects

Cause & Effect
Control
Mastery and pride

Pretend: functional *(12 months)*
Imitation of remembered actions
Use of real objects – pretence mirrors reality

Pretend: symbolic *(18–24 months)*
Linking action with affect
Planning
Narrative structure

Role Play/Social Play
Dramatic play

Figure 3.1 Development of play

No pretence

Pre-symbolic
Brief actions with familiar objects,
eg brings empty cup to mouth
Teasing

Functional pretend
Single pretend actions,
eg brings cup to mouth and
makes drinking action, smiles
Actions are focused on own body

Decoupled pretence
Single pretend actions outside of
present context (deferred imitation),
eg with doll
Single pretend actions which are
normally carried out by other people,
eg driving a car, fighting with a sword

Combined actions
Series of non-sequential pretend actions
with same toys, eg cars and garage
Using one action, eg feeding,
but with different people/toys

Planned pretence
Evidence of advance mental planning,
eg 'I'm going to...'/ 'We're going to be...'
Substitute play objects are more abstract,
showing increased capacity to symbolise
Evidence of a storyline

Figure 3.2 Stages in pretend play

○ The beginning of pretence

The great Russian psychologist Lev Vygotsky provides fascinating insight into how children begin to develop in terms of their ability to pretend. He describes pretend play as a move from the external visual world, where activity is determined purely by the perception of things around, to a more cognitive realm of recollected ideas and internal motives. Vygotsky also notes how, in early pretend play, very little is changed from real life, where a child playing with a doll virtually repeats what his mother does to him. He writes: 'Play is more nearly recollection of something that has actually happened than imagination. It is more memory in action than a novel imaginary situation' (Vygotsky, 1978). He goes on to describe how a child's relation to objects and activities gradually changes as pretend or symbolic play develops. Instead of objects dictating what a child must do – a door to be opened, a staircase to be climbed – increasingly a child's actions in play arise from his ideas about the object. The essence of play development, according to Vygotsky, lies in the fact that a new relation is set up between the visual world and the world of meaning, between real situations and situations in thought.

What is crucial in all of this is the idea of a *staged* development in the child's capacity to pretend. Vygotsky points out that early pretend objects must have properties that suggest the real thing. As he writes, a stick may suggest a horse, but a postcard cannot. These early pretend objects, which he calls 'pivots', serve the function of allowing the child gradually to detach the meaning of 'horse' from a real horse and begin to play with it. In the same way, actions are gradually detached from their real-life meaning as the child closely approximates real actions in pretend situations. The following points from Vygotsky's ideas underpin the activities in this unit:

- early pretence is related to memory
- early substitute objects must have the physical properties of the imagined object
- early pretend actions are almost the same as real actions – pretence is close to mime.

○ Developing pretend play

Some children with autism are able to develop pretend play, though that play does tend to be rigid, repetitive and lacking in complexity and creativity (Cicchetti *et al,* 1994). The social-cognitive deficit that characterises autism means an impairment in the ability to carry out play that includes affect, empathy, cause and effect and sequencing, in other words, the shared cooperative understanding of symbolic play. Children with autism tend to get stuck at the stage of 'functional pretend' play, where pretence is very close to real life and pretend actions tend to be singular rather than combined (Trevarthan *et al,* 1996). In this book, the aim is to identify the skills needed to carry out pretend play and try to address them separately. These skills would include:

- ◉ joint attention
- ◉ shared referencing
- ◉ imitation
- ◉ object substitution
- ◉ mime
- ◉ combining actions with emotion
- ◉ storytelling.

The earlier skills of joint attention, shared referencing and imitation have been discussed in Units 1 and 2, and the skills of combining actions with emotion and/or storytelling will be the focus of Units 6, 7 and 8. This unit concentrates on developing the skills of object substitution and mime, with some more thoughts on imitation. The technique of sculpting will be discussed in the light of how it can be used to develop the use of simple pretence, one that does not involve emotion and does not have a storyline.

Jones (1996) provides a checklist of mimetic skill which is helpful when considering how to build up pretend play. He asks whether the client can do the following:

- mime imaginary objects
- mime physical activities
- mime sensations (feeling cold, hot)
- mime emotions (feeling sad, happy).

All of the above situations could provide the basis for a sculpt. However, it is clear from the checklist that some actions involve the presentation of an outer state only – miming imaginary objects and physical activities – whilst others require the representation of a combined outer state with an inner feeling – miming sensations and actions which express emotion.

The activities

The activities suggested in this unit are concerned only with the outer expression of imagined actions and objects, which are more or less neutral in terms of their emotional content and therefore do not require the consideration of an emotional inner state. The activities concentrate on developing the child's capacity for body and facial expression. The issue of the child's ability to represent things, to imagine objects and to perform pretend actions is also discussed. Activities will range from increasing general body expression to developing a child's capacity to use imaginary objects and carry out imaginary actions, to sculpting proper. Activities will involve mime but the emphasis is on sculpting since, by giving children the opportunity to really look at physical expression, there is the greatest scope for reflection and learning.

Unit 3   Assessment

Area of work | Physical expression & capacity for pretence

Name of child |

Skills	Has this skill	Has demonstrated once in the group	Demonstrates regularly in the group	Has demonstrated outside the group
PHYSICAL EXPRESSION	✓	DATE	DATE	DATE
1 Can create own physical movement or gesture				
2 Can adopt another's movement or gesture, passed on in a circle				
3 Shows flexibility of movement (speed up, slow down, rhythm, high, low)				
4 Uses single parts of the face expressively (eyes widening, mouth opening, eyebrows up and down)				
5 Can show expression through combined use of parts of the face				
6 Allows another to mirror own movements in a pair				
7 Shows consideration for partner when being mirrored				
8 Can mirror with approximation another's movements in a pair				
9 Shows skill, fluency and anticipation of partner when mirroring in a pair				
CAPACITY FOR PRETENCE				
10 Can transform one object into another of similar shape with support				

Unit 3   Assessment *(Continued)*

Skills	Has this skill	Has demonstrated once in the group	Demonstrates regularly in the group	Has demonstrated outside the group
CAPACITY FOR PRETENCE *(Continued)*	✓	DATE	DATE	DATE
11 Can independently transform one object into another of similar shape				
12 Uses body simply to represent a pretend action, with support of a prop (neutral emotion)				
13 Uses body simply to represent a pretend action without use of props (neutral emotion)				
14 Can use body with expression when pretending (combined use of face and parts of body)				
15 Shows appropriate use of space in pretence, outside of usual communicative space				
16 Watches other's pretend actions with interest				
17 Can read other's pretend use of objects and space				
18 Can engage with other's created objects and actions				
19 Enjoys other's and own use of pretence				
20 Can make social inferences based on an individual's use of body				

Notes

____

____

____

Unit 3   Aims

⊙ To develop awareness and expression of the face and body

⊙ To develop the capacity for imitation

⊙ To use imaginary objects and perform simple pretend actions

⊙ To enhance understanding of non-verbal aspects of communication

⊙ To raise peer awareness of the needs of the focus child.

Unit 3   Activities

Mirroring

Mirroring a partner is a key stage in the structured development of a child's ability to adopt certain body postures and carry out specific actions. It is well worth spending time on this activity, familiarising the group with the experience of mirroring and of being mirrored. A mirroring exercise is a useful way of assessing the readiness of the child with autism to take on other people's movements and expression: is he able to copy another child's movements or can he only be copied? This will give a good indication of whether he is ready for the sculpting work that follows.

Both mirroring and performing pretend actions mean adapting one's movements to a situation outside of oneself and require a certain level of body awareness and control. If the child is unable to body mirror, he may respond to further practice on this skill at this stage, but paired with an adult rather than a child. The adult would at first spend time copying the child's body movements and then encourage him to copy her simple movements.

1 Pass the squeeze

This warm-up activity, and the one that follows, may seem a little difficult at first, but children can eventually learn to join in successfully so it is good to persevere.

Instruction

1 With the children sitting in a circle, ask them to hold hands.
2 Tell them that you are going to pass a squeeze around the circle.
3 Tell them that when they feel their hand squeezed they should pass it on by squeezing the hand of the neighbour on their other side.
4 The aim is that the squeeze should eventually go round the circle like a pulse.

Comment

It is possible to see the squeeze going round the circle as children's hands are squeezed. You can point this out to help coordinate the group and achieve a good pace to the activity. For groups that become good at passing the squeeze, tell them to speed up as fast as they can.

2 Pass the gesture

A simple way of copying another person's movements and gestures.

Instruction

1 In a circle, make a gesture and show it to your neighbour who tries to copy it and pass it on.
2 This carries on round the circle until it comes back to the leader.

Variation

Use facial expressions instead of gestures. Although it is hard to avoid expressions that show feelings, that is not the object of the warm-up which should be more in the vein of 'pulling faces' than registering an emotion.

3 Partner mirroring

Body mirroring is a challenging task for a child with autism, who might never be able to copy another person's style of movement. However, for those children who are able to mirror – and some children with autism are very good at it – this is an exercise in adapting oneself to another person.

Instruction

1 In pairs facing each other, instruct one child to copy the other child's movements, as if he is looking in a mirror.
2 Children who are making the lead movements may need some advice on how to move. For example, movement that flows and is not too quick works best.
3 Children who are the mirror image should try to be as precise as possible in following the movement (which is why slow is good), aiming to synchronise their body with that of their partner.
4 After some time, partners swap leader and mirror image roles.

Comment

It does work well to have eye contact during this exercise, but it is not essential. When two children mirror each other, the sense of the other is already quite overwhelming, the movements the other makes absorbed in different ways.

Extension

The activity can be taken further by having the group mirror to music. The mood and power of the movements is enhanced and the exercise becomes highly creative.

4 Hypnosis

This is an Augusto Boal (1992) exercise that children love and is a variation on partner mirroring.

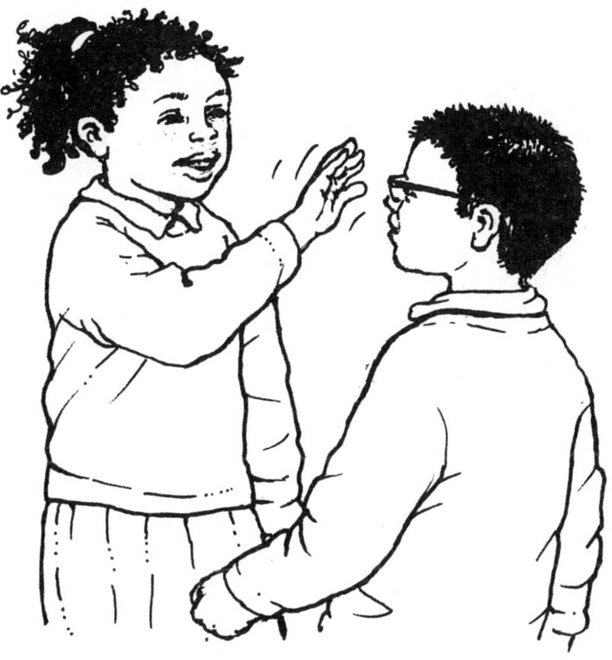

Instruction

1 First explain what it means to hypnotise someone and then give the following instructions.
2 Instead of facing each other, one child (the leader) holds up his hand, palm outwards, a short distance from his partner's face. The hand hypnotises the partner who must follow it, keeping the same distance in between.
3 The leader or hypnotist can now make a series of movements – up, down, right, left, backwards, forwards and diagonal – which the partner follows, contorting their body to keep the right distance from the hand.
4 After a few minutes, tell the partners to swap roles.

5 Moving as one

Children with autism can find this activity difficult at first, but it does require side-by-side rather than face-to-face interaction and can be effective.

Instruction

1 Clear some space and ask the group to line up against a wall at one end of the room.
2 Tell them that they can move across the room, but all together so that no one is obviously leading or lagging behind.
3 Provide a sequence of movements for the group to follow, for example:
   - walking forward three paces
   - turning round
   - walking forward two paces
   - sitting in a row of chairs.
4 Allow the group to first carry out the exercise and then discuss how they did.
5 Practise the sequence a few times so that the children have the opportunity to improve their ability to move as one.

Imaginary objects

The next activities combine the skills of working with objects and using the imagination. This is a crucial stage for a child with autism and it may be necessary to spend time on these activities, regularly repeating them and gradually developing children's skills in this area. Structured pretence is part of all the activities in one of the following ways:

◉ the child is required to imagine something based on a 'pivot' object, that is, a real object that approximates the shape or form of an imagined object (such as a stick to represent a horse).

◉ the activity is first carried out with an actual object and then without the object so that imagining is close to remembering.

6 Popping bubbles

This activity works on the idea of a suggestion of bubbles. The fewer bubbles the better and it is best not to use a bubble gun.

You need

A pot of bubbles.

Instruction

1 Start with actually chasing and popping bubbles, at first blowing real bubbles into the air.
2 Then tell the children that as they move after a bubble they should think about what their arms, hands and face are doing and about their overall direction. Focus their attention by intermittently calling out questions: 'What is your face doing now?', 'Where are your hands?'
3 After a while, the children can be asked to continue to chase a bubble even after it has popped, imagining that it is still there.

Variation

Similar activities would include blowing out a candle, swatting something (a plastic fly on a string) or playing with a yo-yo. Objects should be ephemeral, something that is there but not solidly there.

7 Transform the object

In this activity, children use pivot objects similar in size and shape to the imagined object.

You need

Three objects of roughly the same shape but different size, such as a cocktail stick, a chopstick and a metre rule.

Instruction

1 Taking each object in turn, starting with the smallest, pass it round the circle asking the children to transform it into something else. Each child needs to mime an action with the object, for example, using the cocktail stick as a sewing needle or the metre rule as a sword.
2 The group should guess what the imagined object is.

Comment

The idea of the exercise is that the imagined object should not be that different from the actual object, and children with autism usually find this exercise straightforward. The change in size, however, helps to develop imagination and lateral thinking. Different shaped objects can be used but it is a good idea to keep to basic shapes such as circles, rings, spheres, cubes and cylinders.

8 Objects in nature

Natural objects with interesting shapes and textures make good pivot objects for imaginative work.

You need

Natural objects such as pebbles, leaves, a branch, driftwood, shells and a camera.

Instruction

1 Combine some of the objects to represent something else in nature: the pebbles and leaves to make a nest; the branch standing upright to represent a tree. Ask the children to think of their own ideas.
2 Take photographs of the objects that the children create, stick them into a book and record each: 'Ben used pebbles and leaves to make a pretend nest.'

Variation

Found objects are also good for making faces, arranging objects to make eyes, nose and a mouth. As children with autism begin to be able to represent things,

I find that they often become fascinated with drawing faces. All kinds of different faces can be made and, again, photographs taken for a book of faces.

9 The imaginary ball

In this activity, the imaginative work is based on something real that happened very recently and is therefore easy to recall.

You need

A selection of balls of different colour, size and weight.

Instruction

1 With the children standing in a circle, throw a soft ball around the group until they become familiar with the act of catching and throwing.
2 Take the ball away and ask the children to pretend to throw and catch it.
3 Repeat the activity, varying the size and weight of the ball and each time doing a real round of catching and throwing followed by an imaginary round.
4 Tell the children to think about what they are doing with their hands, body and face when they catch a large, light ball as opposed to a small, heavy ball and ask them to try to replicate this when they pretend to do the same action.

Comment

Many children with autism have motor difficulty and find it hard to perform actions that involve catching and throwing. This activity may not be suitable for them, but you might consider simply passing the ball or using easy to catch balls (there is now a selection commercially available, see Useful Contacts on p216).

10 Handling imaginary objects

Requiring a little more in terms of pretence, children must express an imagined object more fully.

You need

Objects that are interesting in terms of their shape, size and weight, and that contrast with each other in some way. Examples would be a floor cushion, a large empty box, a tiny bead, something sticky and a plate of marbles.

Instruction

1 Pass each object around the circle, again asking the children to be aware of their face, hands and body as they do so.

2 Take the object away and ask the group to repeat the exercise, now imagining that object.

3 When a few objects have been tried and the group, including the focus child, can pass an imaginary object convincingly, ask individuals to choose one of the objects and pretend to handle it while the rest of the group try to guess what it is.

Comment

Some people with autism are hypersensitive and find the feel of some textures unpleasant, so it is important to select items carefully.

Extension

Repeat the exercise of passing an imaginary object. As the children do this, look out for good examples of face and body expression and ask that person to freeze as if they have become a statue. Tell the rest of the group to go and look at the statue, moving round it and noticing the face, hands and different parts of the body. Use the sculpt as a teaching resource, pointing out what the hands, face, legs and feet are doing and how that conveys the impression of carrying something. Ask the circle to re-form and copy the posture of the statue. Do this a few times, choosing different children each time.

Pretend actions

Although the previous activities using imaginary objects do involve actions, basing the pretence on the use of an object means the presence of a strong real or remembered element. The following activities are simply about 'doing something' and probably require more in the way of imaginative work.

11 Washing

A warm-up for the face and body, getting the children ready for work on physical expression.

Instruction

1 Ask the children to wash their faces and clean their teeth, demonstrating the actions of rubbing the face and brushing teeth.
2 If it is inappropriate to introduce an imaginative element at this stage, tell the children simply to gently massage their faces.
3 Care should be taken to include all the areas of the face so that children get a sense of their whole face.

Extension

Take the idea further by having a bath. Sit down and rub all the parts of the body, as if washing in a bath.

12 Chewing

This involves another simple pretend action of putting food in the mouth and chewing it.

Instruction

1 Demonstrate a chewing action, making chewing actions and noises with your mouth and jaws.
2 If you want to take the imaginary element further, specify what you are eating, for example, sipping soup or chewing a sticky toffee.

Variation

Try chewing bubblegum and blowing bubbles, the hands indicating the size of it, until it is huge. When it pops, pull the imaginary bubble stickily off the face.

13 What am I doing?

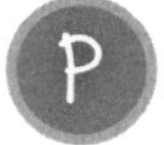

In this simple exercise the group leader mimes an activity and the group guesses what he is doing. It is important to choose the activity well. Good ideas are ones with which the children are familiar and that can be mimed simply.

You need

Mime ideas (p203).

Instruction

1 Decide on a mime and show it to the group.
2 Ask the children to guess what it is you are doing.
3 Children take turns to be leader but consider carefully whether you want them to decide on their own mimes. You may find they can mime more successfully if you provide the idea.

Variation

It is possible to do the above activity as a group. One child leaves the room whilst the others agree on a mime. All the group members do the mime together. The individual who left returns, watches the mime and guesses the activity.

14 Action mirrors

This activity combines mirroring and pretence.

Instruction

1 Working in pairs, ask one child to be leader and the other to copy him, as in mirrored partner work.
2 Ask the lead child to mime something (or give him an activity to mime). See Mime ideas (p203) for some suggestions.
3 The other child should try to copy his actions as precisely as possible, as a mirror image.
4 After the pairs have mirrored each other for a while, ask the mirror child to say what it was he was miming.

15 Sculpt an action

This is similar to the previous activity, but requires a little more skill in terms of imagination and physical expression.

Instruction

1 In pairs, ask one child to be a 'sculptor' and think of an action, and the other child to be the 'model'.
2 The sculptor makes his sculpture, telling his model what to do, demonstrating the action to be performed and moulding the arms, legs, body, hands and face appropriately.
3 The sculptor spends a little time watching the sculpt in action, making sure the movements are right and tweaking if necessary.
4 The sculptor then brings his sculpt to life for the group to watch.

Extension

The activity can become a 'Twenty Questions' exercise, with the group guessing the action being performed by directing questions to the sculptor, to which he can only answer yes or no.

16 Abstract sculpts

This is an enjoyable exercise, but it is abstract and so may not be appropriate for some children who need concrete, reality-based stimulus. However, some children enjoy sound and movement and may really take to the activity.

You need

Movement and sound words (p204).

Instruction

1 Ask the group to form pairs with one child as sculptor and the other as model.
2 The sculptor moulds his model into a particular pose by moving his arms, legs and head.
3 He gives his sculpt a movement and a sound by choosing one word to describe a movement and one to describe a sound.
4 Once he is happy with his sculpt, he can show it to the rest of the group. The rest of the group can ask the sculptor what it is he has made: person, animal, machine or monster, though children may prefer that no particular social meaning is imposed on their sculpture.

The final element of this unit uses sculpting in its most traditional form, that is, as a way of representing social scenes and social relationships. However, at this stage, work will concentrate on only the physical aspects of a social scene – for example, orientation, proximity, gesture and eye contact – rather than any emotional or verbal content. Sculpts require the group to consider what happens physically between two people when they relate. The task for the group is to look for clues that indicate what the pair's relationship might be and to practise those aspects of social interaction.

An interesting example of the use of sculpted scenes comes from fourteenth-century Central Asia where simple drawn scenes, or cartoons, showing two people in relation to each other, were used as a springboard for oral storytelling. Two or more people would be depicted 'in relation', standing near to one another, oriented towards each other in some way, or one engaged in a task and the other watching or indicating something. The form reached its peak in the work of the artist known as Mohammed of the Black Pen who painted simple yet beautiful and highly expressive social scenes. They do not tell a particular story and have no allegorical element, but simply show something going on between two people. The story that followed was meant to fill in the missing pieces of the puzzle, the depictions being loose enough to allow any number of possible stories.

These next activities use the idea of frozen depictions of non-specific social situations, to encourage the group to contemplate what happens physically between two people when they are relating, and to speculate on what might be happening between them.

17 Sculpting social scenes 1

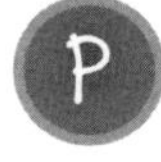 A powerful way of learning about social situations which can be done in the safety of a group. This activity gives children ample time to observe and think about what might be going on between two or more people.

You need

Illustrations of different social scenes (see Scene cards on pp205–6).

Instruction

1 Choose a scene from the cards and select the right number of children needed to sculpt it. Ask the remainder of the group to form an audience.

2 Tell the children to replicate the scene showing the same orientation, distance from each other, posture, gesture and facial expression as the figures in the illustration.

3 Instruct the audience to contemplate the sculpt, noticing such details as face, hands, body, proximity and direction they are facing. They may walk around it if they wish to view it from different angles.

4 Ask the question, 'Who are these people and what are they doing?'

5 Elicit a number of responses to demonstrate the fact that there could be more than one answer to this question and so encourage flexibility of thought.

18 Sculpting social scenes 2

This exercise takes the activity a little further.

You need

Illustrations of different social scenes (see Scene cards, pp205–6).

Instruction

1 Choose a scene from the cards and select the right number of children needed to sculpt it. Ask the remainder of the group to form an audience.

2 Tell the children to replicate the scene showing the same orientation, distance from each other, posture, gesture and facial expression as the figures in the illustration.

3 Go into the scene deeper by labelling the sculpt characters A, B, C and ask questions about each in turn:
  - What is A doing with his face, body, hands, eyes?
  - How are A and B standing in relation to each other?
  - Who do you think will speak first and why?
  - What might he say?
  - What might happen next?
  - What do you think is going on between these two or more people?

Comment

At this stage, avoid questions about how characters feel. Later on, sculpting exercises can be used to think about expression, actions and feeling.

Extension

Alter one thing in the sculpt by changing an orientation or adding a gesture or another character, and ask what might be happening now.

19 What's wrong?

Similar to the previous activity, here children are asked to think about something that is not right in terms of body language, orientation and proximity.

Instruction

1 One person, adult or child, sculpts a scene using other group members. It should be of an ordinary everyday event with which people are familiar.
2 One element should be included that is clearly out of place in a scene such as this.
3 The audience have to guess the content of the scene and point out what is wrong with it.

Comment

This activity can be used to teach awareness of right and wrong places to touch someone to get their attention.

20 Distance-o-meter

This activity experiments with a child's preference in terms of the proximity of other people.

Instruction

1 Ask one child to stand in the middle of the room and another to stand opposite at one end.
2 Have the second person approach the first slowly.
3 The first should say 'Stop' when he feels this person is at a comfortable distance.
4 Try out different ways of approach, asking which feels most comfortable each time. Examples to compare would be:
    - approaching from the front, approaching from behind and approaching from the side
    - approaching from the front making eye contact and not making eye contact
    - talking at a distance and talking at very close quarters
    - the first person blindfolded and the second stopping at different distances and speaking.

Comment

Freezing and sculpting can be used to raise other children's awareness of how people with autism may prefer alternative forms of physical relating to non-autistic people. Ways of relating that are thought correct by non-autistic people, such as making eye contact, standing close and touching, may only be correct for people who do not have autism. A person with autism may prefer a different way of relating physically that does not include any of these things.

Introduction

The use of a script – a set of verbal statements that are memorised and rehearsed – is common in work with autism. The generation of language in children with autism is a key issue, and one way to overcome the difficulty is to provide a ready-made language, in the form of given sentences. The aim is to teach these statements to the child so that he uses them in appropriate social situations. Children with autism can learn set phrases, for example, for greeting people and saying goodbye, or for asking for and naming things. The Lovaas method uses this approach, requiring 'verbal imitation' from a child, the repetition of set phrases for which he is rewarded (Trevarthan *et al*, 1996). Through this conditioning, the child learns to perform certain behaviours, including speech, in certain situations. Language programmes based on this approach employ strategies such as providing the beginnings of set sentences which the child is asked to complete, as in 'My name is ___' and 'I like to play with ___'.

Some script-based work with children with autism, however, takes more of a developmental approach, assuming that the child will increasingly internalise the language he is being provided with. Pamela Wolfberg, in her Integrated Play Group, explains how she writes out verbal cues for the children in the group, telling them exactly what to say to another child during a play interaction. She found that all three children with whom she worked developed, though to different degrees, and this included a general improvement in their spoken language (Wolfberg, 1999). The Picture Exchange Communication System (PECS), developed by Lori Frost and Andy Bondy and used so successfully in work with autism, is also at heart a script-based approach. After initial exchanges of symbols for desired objects, children are expected to make up sentences using prefixes such as 'I want ___' or 'I see ___', and then read them or complete the ending. Though the aim of the programme is the promotion of skill in communication, it has been found that at the sentence-building stage children tend also to develop their capacity for more spontaneous speech (Baker, 2000; Cumine *et al*, 2000).

Social communication programmes, not specifically designed for use with children with autism, but popularly used to develop their language, tend also to contain components of work that involve scripted encounters in social situations (Rinaldi, 1992; Schroeder, 1997).

⭘ The cultural 'scripts' of childhood

Scripts are actually important for all children, an aspect of children's culture in general. There are the songs, finger rhymes and simple word games learned in early childhood, such as 'Row the boat' or 'See you later, alligator', that could be loosely described as 'scripts'. There is also the 'lore and language' that children pass on to each other. Historically, children have always used given rhymes, riddles, jokes and insults, learned from other children and adopted as their own. The sheer accumulation of such sayings is wonderfully encapsulated in the work of Peter and Iona Opie, who describe how children learn verbal pieces by heart and transmit them over several generations without corruption (Opie & Opie, 1959).

The ability to make sense is definitely not a requirement of these childhood scripts. However, such things as rhyme, rhythm and repetition, as well as a certain back and forth quality that suggests sociability and interaction, are essential characteristics. It is the liveliness and playfulness of the lines that are the overriding features: their 'oomph and zoom' and ability to 'pack a punch' (Opie & Opie, 1992).

Such social exchange is appropriate for children with autism too. The literature recommends songs and other social routines to develop a child's capacity for interaction and communication in general (Cumine *et al*, 2000; Hannah, 2001; Moor, 2002). One category of children's lore that lends itself to developing speech in particular in a child with autism could be broadly designated as 'repartee' and would concern the type of songs and sayings that involve call and response. These are truly scripts, in the sense that they are made up of a number of given lines which are spoken by two or more people.

⭘ Using call and response

Examples of call and response include such songs as 'Ten in the bed' and 'Old MacDonald had a farm', where individuals must provide a line before the song can continue. In the first instance, the line is given – 'Roll over, roll over' – but in the second, the child must think of his own response, in this instance, the name of a farmyard animal. For a child with autism, though he may enjoy both types of song, it is easier to participate in the first than in the second type, where he may need prompting by being given the name of an animal. In fact, the structure of 'Ten in the bed' gives the illusion that the child is interacting *himself*, without any adult mediation, even though it is a strictly learned response.

There are some versions of call and response that may be more problematic for a child with autism. Songs that stay on imaginatively neutral or safe ground are fine, but some songs stray into riskier realms. For a child with autism, who may have a disordered sense of what is real and what is not real, repartee like 'What's the time, Mr Wolf?' may be a little too frightening. For the same tone of excited anticipation, 'Here is a beehive' (see Call and response songs and rhymes, pp86–8) would be a good alternative.

○ Using the voice

Any work on speech requires preliminary work on developing the voice and vocal expression. For many children with autism, their voice is characteristic of their condition. Some children have a very small quiet voice, some use little expression and have a flat monotone voice, some produce their voice in the throat only so that their speech sounds slightly strangulated. Some children with autism speak with an accent, often an American-sounding accent, or use different accents.

The voice is close to personality and is part of who we are. This is also true of people with autism. It is proposed here that, before any work on vocal expression is begun, careful consideration should be given to why it is felt necessary to develop and therefore change a child's voice. In other words, the reason should not simply be that it sounds 'unpleasant' or 'not right' in some way, since the problem here clearly lies with the listener rather than the child.

Sometimes it is appropriate to do work on vocal expression, for example, with a child who is talking in a forced way and therefore straining his vocal muscles. Children can be helped to use more of their voice as well as to use a bigger voice, which can assist them in their communication and general capacity for social interaction. Voice work is an enjoyable way of working, good for building group awareness and helping to make a group gel together. It is playful and expressive and can contribute, incidentally, to the development of a child's self-esteem and personality.

Chloe, aged nine, talked little and when she did she put her hand over her mouth and used a small voice. She would talk only to one or two people, adults with whom she was familiar, and refused to talk at all to others, particularly adults in authority.

In weekly small group work, activities were used to help build trust and a sense of safety, with the same few children who did not have autism and were socially mature working with Chloe each time. After a while, exercises focused on using the voice to make sounds as well as speech. There was an emphasis on activities being playful and fun, with the same exercises being used over again to establish a safe sense of predictability. Chloe enjoyed the weekly sessions. After a few months, her voice became less strangulated and monotone, sounding louder, `bigger' and more confident. She became more generally assertive and playful in her manner, contributing creative ideas of her own and generating more language spontaneously. Her support worker started to sit away from her in the group since Chloe no longer required the same level of prompting.

Unit 4   Assessment

Area of work | *Vocal expression & use of a script*

Name of child |

Skills	Has this skill	Has demonstrated once in the group	Demonstrates regularly in the group	Has demonstrated outside the group
VOCAL EXPRESSION	✓	DATE	DATE	DATE
1 Can produce own sound independently				
2 Can vocalise another person's sound				
3 Can coordinate vocal expression with others in a group				
4 Can make a variety of sounds				
5 Shows flexibility in vocal expression and strength (loud, quiet, fast, slow, rhythmic)				
6 Can use voice to represent pretend material				
USE OF A SCRIPT				
7 Can use set lines in a call and response situation				
8 Can generate a new line in a call and response situation				
9 Can use a selection of given non-verbal greetings				
10 Can use a selection of given verbal greetings				

Unit 4   Assessment *(Continued)*

Skills	Has this skill	Has demonstrated once in the group	Demonstrates regularly in the group	Has demonstrated outside the group
USE OF A SCRIPT *(Continued)*	✓	DATE	DATE	DATE
11 Can use a scripted line in structured situations/series				
12 Can say a scripted line with proper emphasis and expression				
13 Can take part in a short scripted conversation with a familiar person				
14 Can adopt appropriate body posture, orientation and distance in structured situations				
15 Can take part in a short scripted conversation with an unfamiliar person				
16 Can generate own language, based on a rehearsed script, in conversation				

Notes

____

____

____

____

____

____

____

____

- ◎ To raise awareness of the rhythms of conversation and develop skills in turn taking

- ◎ To develop vocal strength and expression

- ◎ To create, rehearse and role play scripts to develop child's everyday conversations.

Unit 4   Activities

<u>**Call and response songs and rhymes**</u>

Songs and rhymes that use call and response provide a preliminary stage to working with a script based on the child's own daily experience of conversation. Initially, work can be done just on call and response, providing a bridge between the stage of singing together and that of talking together. In fact, some songs lend themselves to being converted into a call and response situation and can be adapted instead of being sung.

Here are some examples of call and response for use with individuals and groups. Individual responses are written in italics.

1 Here is a beehive

Children love this rhyme. It is done with an action accompaniment of hands slotted together with the fingers facing down and wriggling as if they are the bees.

ADULT Here is a beehive
CHILD But where are all the bees?
ADULT They're hiding inside where nobody sees
       Here they come creeping, out of the door
       1-2-3-4
       Buzzzz

The opening of the door is indicated by the thumbs opening up, and the counting is accompanied by each finger – index, middle, ring and little finger – joining at the tip and opening up the hands. *'Buzzz'* takes the form of tickling the children. The responder has only one line, which need not be the whole line and could be simply *'Bees?'*, though some children like to count out the '1-2-3-4' as well.

2 Who stole the cookie from the cookie jar?

This is a perfect example of call and response and gives a very good approximation of an actual conversation.

ADULT Who stole the cookie from the cookie jar?
       Did you steal the cookie from the cookie jar? [*point at one individual*]
CHILD Who, me? [*pointing at self*]
ADULT Yes, you [*pointing again with emphasis*]
CHILD Couldn't have been [*shaking head*]
ADULT Then who? [*opening out hands in questioning gesture*]
CHILD Jake [*naming and pointing at another group member*]

ADULT Did you steal the cookies from the cookie jar? *[song continues – pointing at next child]*

The elements of pointing a finger and shaking the head are interesting in that they are not straightforward ones for children with autism and may need some work.

3 Knock, knock

Although it appears to be simple, 'Knock, knock' is a deceptively difficult script since the child who knocks often wants to say 'Who's there?' as well. For children with autism, who have a weak grasp of the reciprocity of subject and object ('me then you') this script can be doubly tricky, but well worth the effort.

ADULT Knock, knock
CHILD Who's there?
ADULT Sarah
CHILD Sarah who?
ADULT Sarah Brown

The adult takes the 'Knock, knock' role first, giving one half and then the other half of her name and so models the lines. The child would first need to learn the script, 'Who's there?'/'Sarah who?' Later it may be possible to reverse the roles, with the child doing the knocking.

4 Garden path

This is a memory rhyme with partners taking it in turn to say what they have seen along the garden path, adding a new one each time. It does require the child to provide some ideas of his own, that is, what he saw along the path, though responses can be prompted. Its use of 'my/your' is interesting for the alternation of subject and object and is a nice way of teaching this aspect of language and social understanding.

ADULT/CHILD I went down the garden path today
ADULT/CHILD And what did you see along the way?
ADULT/CHILD I saw my tree, your flower, my cat, your...

Take turns in beginning the rhyme, so that the subject alternates between you and the child. For children who are having difficulty with this, use a visual prompt that they can hold. Two stones with the words *'my'* and *'your'* painted on may be used, for example. The child and his partner (adult or another child) hold the stone that is correct for the part they are about to speak, 'my' for the person saying the first line and 'your' for the responder. Stones can be tapped, indicating the correct word usage, to reinforce that part of the script. When roles are reversed, the stones can be swapped over as a physical and visual indication of the changeover of the 'me' and 'you' roles.

5 Tick tock

This activity is done in a group with the object being passed from person to person around the circle. The object should go all the way round and back to the leader.

ADULT   This is a tick *[offering pen or other object to neighbour on the right]*
CHILD   A what?
ADULT   A tick
CHILD   *[takes the object, turns to neighbour and starts again]* This is a tick

When the group is able to use the script, take another object similar to the first but distinguishable in some way (eg two pens of different colour), and pass that to your neighbour on the left. This time the script is:

ADULT   This is a tock
CHILD   A what?
ADULT   A tock

When this object has been passed round the circle successfully, you can send both tick and tock off in different directions. One child will have to negotiate both objects as they pass across each other, which is a good exercise in turn taking and having to order your communication.

6 Hello, hello, hello, sir

This is a traditional skipping song and so has a satisfying rhythm.

ADULT   Hello, hello, hello, sir
           Meet me at the grocer
CHILD   No, sir
ADULT   Why, sir?
CHILD   Because I have a cold, sir
ADULT   Where did you get your cold, sir?
CHILD   At the North Pole, sir
ADULT   What were you doing there, sir?
CHILD   Counting polar bears, sir
ADULT   Let me hear you sneeze, sir
CHILD   Aitchoo, aitchoo, aitchoo

The rhyme is long and harder to learn but may be suitable for children who are really beginning to use their voices. Have some fun with the sneezing at the end.

Activities for working with the voice

The idea here is that a child can be 'woken up' to his voice and made more aware of it by having it reflected back by another person or by the group. Of course, for children who are hypersensitive to sound, care should be taken that things do not get too loud.

7 Echoes

This activity uses the familiar idea of 'mirroring' the child with autism, but this time using the voice and sound rather than the body and movement.

You need

A volume gauge (p207) and a badge.

Instruction

1 In a circle, one person is asked to be leader and given a badge to indicate this (eg a badge with a star). The leader makes a sound which the group echoes back. The echo should be longer than the initial sound and can reverberate a little as in a real echo.
2 Help to coordinate the echo by using a countdown '3-2-1' or 'Ready, steady, go'.
3 Encourage the echo to build in volume by using the volume gauge as a visual prompt. You can run your finger along the gauge, indicating that the group should get louder or quieter, or point at the gauge to show how loud the echo should be.
4 Use the same sound a few times or, if more creativity is possible, change the sound each time there is a new leader.

8 Echo partners

Instead of making echoes as a whole group, create echoes in pairs.

Instruction

1 Put the children into pairs and ask them to face each other.
2 Give them a long tube to hold between them.
3 One person makes a sound into the tube which is placed at their partner's ear. Care should be taken that the sound is not too loud or the tube too close to the ear since sound is concentrated in this way.
4 The partner then echoes back the sound through the tube in the same way.

9 Volume control

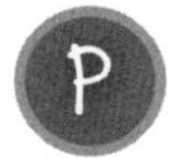

This activity is designed to increase the quantity of sound a child can produce.

You need

A set sentence, perhaps one taken from the call and response songs and rhymes (see pp86–8) and the volume gauge (p207).

Instruction

1 Practise the sentence with the group using different volumes, using the volume gauge.
2 Combine volume and distance by dividing the group and having them face each other across the room.
3 Experiment with different volumes at different distances.
4 Use a conflicting volume/distance ratio, for example, whispering at a distance or shouting up close, and ask the group for feedback about how this feels.

Variation

It is possible to do the whole activity as a call and response exercise, with the group divided and facing each other. Give the subgroups a line each – 'See you later, alligator/In a while, crocodile' – and have them call to each other and respond. Encourage vocal expression by turning the group volume up and down.

10 Orchestra

This activity develops the quality and expression of the voice.

You need

Different musical instruments that make a variety of interesting sounds.

Instruction

1 Play each instrument to the group.
2 Using suggestions from the group, transform the sound produced by the instrument into a vocal sound.
3 Ask each child to choose the instrument they are going to become and ask them to practise their sound.
4 One person, acting as a conductor and possibly holding a baton, stands in front of the group who are now lined up like an orchestra. The conductor conducts by pointing to people to make their sound.

5 Discuss how a conductor uses different gestures to control an orchestra. Suggest that children use these to get two people to play at the same time, to keep one instrument going while bringing in others or to change the volume of sound.

A script is a set of spoken words, a dialogue that is written down. In work with autism, this immediately raises a question: whose words do we use? It is not always possible to ask the child in question, who is using little speech, to provide the ideas for a scripted conversation. So whose ideas can we use?

The group of non-autistic children amongst whom the child with autism is learning is a valuable resource here. I have found that, typically, the best scripts with the liveliest and most authentic feeling lines are in fact those generated by children. Language may not be grammatical or even always make sense, but the feel of the language will be much better than that produced by an adult or found in a book.

The best method of generating and recording ideas for a script is a circle time approach combined with the activity of brainstorming.

11 Brainstorm

Use a small circle of children, which includes the child with autism who is the focus of the group, and brainstorm a script around one aspect of the school day.

You need

Large sheets of paper and a pen.

Instruction

1. Choose a time of day or particular situation that is socially difficult, such as playtimes or interacting with teachers. Talk to the group about what typically happens at that time.
2. If the script is to concern personal material, such as talking to friends, it is possible to talk about the personality of the child in question. Ask the group to think positively about his attributes: his abilities, what he does and does not like to do, and so on.
3. Have the children brainstorm things they say at that time or to that person.
4. Write down the children's statements verbatim until the paper is full.
5. Read back the lines to the group and say you will bring them back for more work when they have been typed.
6. In typing up the children's statements, you may want to edit them a little, for example, to reduce any sense of repetition or to increase the meaning

of the line. However, lines should have a lively quality and need not be grammatically correct.

Comment

An important aspect of scripts is that they have a written element. People with autism often prefer ways of communicating that are not person to person and verbal, and writing may be a preferred alternative. The fact that scripts are initially in a written form can be used to great advantage in work with children with autism. Part of the development of the work and of the child should involve a managed transition from the written word to the spoken word. Some children may manage that transition well, some may need it to be structured, and others may not manage it at all or only with a continued need for prompting.

examples of scripts for the school day

Talking to the teacher

Excuse me, miss
I want help
Is it playtime yet?
I want the toilet
I want a drink
Is it lunchtime yet?
I'm finished. What do I do now?
I don't want help, thank you
Is it home time?
Someone is annoying me

Lunchtime

I want to sit with you
Do you want to sit with me?
Look, I've got sandwiches, crisps, yoghurt and a biscuit
What's in your box?
I like to drink water
What do you like to drink?
Is your lunch nice?
Me too?
Shall we go out to play?
Let's go!

Playing

Want to play?
I like running games
I chase you, you chase me
What games do you like?
Do you want to play ball?
Stand over there
I throw the ball to you
Ready, steady, go
You throw the ball to me
Do you want a race?
Ready, steady, go

Talking to a friend

My name's _______
What's your name?
I've got a train set and computer games
What toys have you got?
Look, I've got this
I like watching videos
What videos have you got?
Do you like singing?
Can you come to my house for tea?
Do you want to play with me?
Let's run!

Learning the lines

In order to be successful, work with scripts needs to be highly structured and controlled. It is recommended, in fact, that the following activities are carried out in order, following the instruction closely. The first two activities serve as warm-ups for learning the lines; the following three move into learning the lines that have been generated in a group brainstorm (see Activity 11 above).

As a preliminary to working with the scripted lines produced by the group, you will need to write out the script clearly or type it. For young children or children who have difficulty with reading, write out the statements adding pictures for key words. Cut out the statements so that there is one statement per strip of paper. For the rehearsal session, sit the group on chairs in a circle.

12 Chair swaps

Get the children used to moving in and out of chairs and meeting other children in the circle whilst remembering a piece of information.

Instruction

1 Stand in the middle of the circle and call out the names of two group members.
2 They must try to swap seats whilst the person in the middle tries to sit down on one of their empty chairs.
3 Whoever is left standing calls out another two names.

Extension

Extend this activity by requiring children to remember information as they move around the circle. Give a child an item in a category. For example, if the category is 'fruit', group members choose to become an apple, banana, melon, and so on. Children must remember the item they have become as well as other group members' items. Standing in the middle of the circle, call out the names of two fruit. These two children should then swap chairs while you try to sit in one of them. Whoever is left standing calls out another two items.

Comment

Children with autism have difficulty with the concept of categories but I find that simple straightforward ones usually work. Try colours, items of clothing or furniture.

13 Greetings

Another warm-up activity that introduces a more social element.

Instruction

1 Ask the children for ideas on how we greet each other non-verbally, for example, shaking hands, bowing, smiling.
2 Demonstrate their suggestions and instruct them to choose one method, keeping it to themselves.
3 Call out the names of two people who go into the circle to meet. They greet each other in one of these ways and then sit in each other's seats.
4 Children can take it in turn to be the leader.

Variation

Do the same as above, thinking of what we say when we greet each other verbally.

14 Memorising the lines

 Begin to use the scripts that the group have generated in their brainstorm.

You need

One line of script, written out, per child.

Instruction

1 Give each child one written line to say. Go through it with them to check for understanding.
2 Sitting in a circle, point to children who must then read out their statement.
3 This exercise should speed up as the group members become familiar with their statement.
4 Eventually, as statements are memorised, papers can be discarded and lines simply spoken.

15 Encouraging expression

Start to play with the lines, to increase the children's familiarity with them and to bring a sense of playfulness and expression to the work.

Instruction

1 Ask the children to:
    ◎ whisper their statement to the person sitting on the right
    ◎ pass a ball across the circle saying the line
    ◎ standing in a line along one end of the room, sing out their line like an opera singer, trying to fill the space in front of them
    ◎ one child can be asked to stand in the middle of the circle and speak the line with group members joining him in turn, speaking their line as they come into the centre.

16 Beginning to interact

Begin to interact by using the warm-up activity of two people meeting in the middle of the circle.

Instruction

1 Call out two names, and as the two people meet ask them to speak their lines to each other.
2 These two sit down and another two names are called, so that the same lines are used in different combinations.

Comment

As a way of giving the lines more sense conversationally, it is possible to specify who should speak first and who second. However, it is not essential that the dialogue makes absolute sense. Lines could be, for example:

FIRST CHILD	Is your lunch nice?
SECOND CHILD	Look I've got sandwiches and a biscuit
FIRST CHILD	What games do you like?
SECOND CHILD	Do you want to play ball?

The idea of the work is to give an approximation of conversation, the *feel* of a spoken interaction between two people, its physical back and forth quality, liveliness and how it relates to a subject that both participants know about. After all, real-life conversations can be disjointed and may not always flow or make proper sense.

Once the scripts have been memorised and rehearsed, they can be used as the basis for a role play. However, for a child with autism who is at this stage of social communication, working with role play needs to be as structured as the rehearsal work that has gone before. Role play is a powerful way of working, particularly for a child who has a disordered sense of what real life is, and work should always be carefully thought through.

As with the previous exercises, it is important to build up the children's capacity to role play scripts in the following sequence of activities.

17 The empty chair

Use a classic drama technique that does not require actual interaction with another person.

You need

Scripted lines, one per child.

Instruction

1 Have the group sit in an open-ended circle with an empty chair placed in the gap.
2 Children take turns to approach the empty chair, speak or read their line to the chair, as if someone is sitting there, and then sit down.
3 The next child then approaches, until all children have spoken their lines.

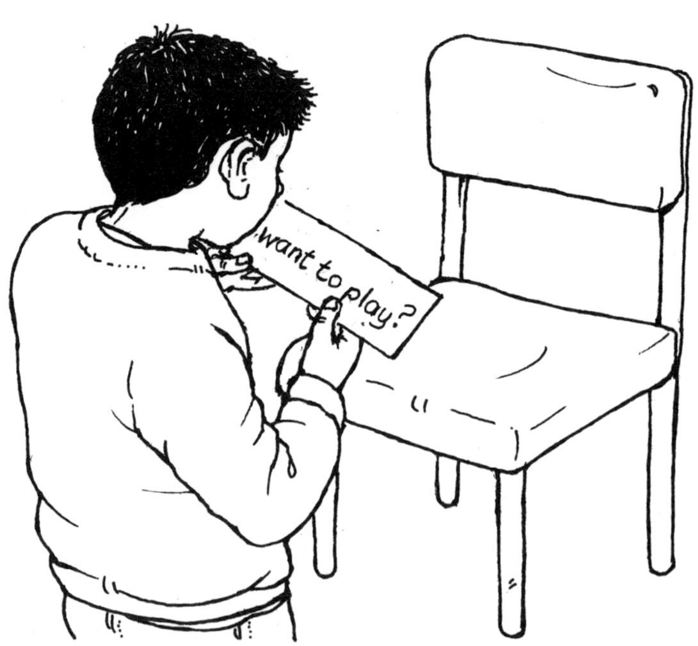

18 A child 'in role'

This activity gradually introduces another person into the role play by having a child who does not actually speak sit in the chair.

Instruction

1 One child, probably a non-autistic child, sits on the previously empty chair 'in role'. This means adopting the role of one participant in the scripted conversation, for example, the teacher or a friend.
2 The other children, including the child with autism, go up to the child in role and speak their line. The child in role need not reply though he may want to respond non-verbally in some way.

19 Incorporating structure in the role play

Some children with autism may find Activity 18, instructing them to interact with another child in role, too difficult since, role play or not, it is actually requiring them to communicate. You may need to introduce more structure to enable them to carry out the task.

Instruction

1 Provide extra prompts as you carry out the activity of a child in role sitting in the chair, which might include:
    - the child with autism giving his written line to the child in role to read
    - the child with autism reading his written script to the child sitting in the chair
    - directly prompting the child by speaking the first few words of his line and pausing for the child to complete the line.

20 Combining scripts with scenes

Choose depictions of scenes that best fit the children's scripts from the selection of Scene cards (see pp205–6).

Instruction

1 Taking each scene in turn, ask one child to sculpt the scene using other group members, the remainder of the group becoming the audience.
2 The sculpt should show proximity, body posture, gesture and facial expression, but nothing should be said at this stage. Just ask the audience to observe the sculpt.

Comment

The audience can watch the sculpts brought to life in the following ways:

- You read from some of the scripts as the children take part in the sculpt.
- You give the participants a line each to say, maybe the line or lines they have already used in the rehearsals and role play. You or a member of the audience can put a hand on the shoulder of one of the sculpt participants, who should then speak his line.
- One person acting as director can call 'Action' and bring the sculpt to life, the participants speaking their lines in turn and then freezing again.

Making everyday use of scripts

Scripts produced and rehearsed in a small group can be taken into and used in everyday life. With some children, this happens spontaneously, simply developing their use of one-word statements to longer and more complex sentences whilst making greater use of their voices. For other children, however, the transition may need to be managed so that the child is required to build up his use of speech in a structured way. The following is a possible transition plan from small group work to everyday usage, with the emphasis throughout being 'one thing at a time'. More support can be provided for the child if the communicative partner is an adult.

○ First stage: communication partners reading lines

A single communicative partner, a time of day or an event is identified. Then the child is given the appropriate sentence for the situation. Examples might be:

CHILD TO A TEACHER   I've finished my work. What shall I do now?
CHILD AT LUNCHTIME   I'd like this for my dinner and that for pudding *[pointing to choice]*

Lines are written down for both the child and his conversation partner (parent, teacher, auxiliary staff, another child). The conversation is read by each in turn. The emphasis here should not be on eye contact or correct body orientation. The sole focus should be on taking turns to say the words of the script.

○ Second stage: child only reading line

The child only reads his line, with his conversation partner responding more spontaneously. At this point, he can be encouraged to face towards and look at his partner when he has finished reading his line.

○ Third stage: speak memorised and rehearsed lines

The conversation takes place using set lines, but ones that are *spoken* and not read. Rehearsed lines should be adhered to with no encouragement at this point for greater spontaneity or flexibility. The aim of this stage of the work is getting the child used to the physical intimacy of a spoken conversation where two people are facing each other.

○ Final stage: child has a repertoire of conversational lines

The child takes part in a conversation choosing what to say from two or three given lines that have been worked on, memorised and rehearsed previously, in small group time.

Props, Puppets, Costume 
Exploring objects and people as objects

Introduction

There can be no doubt that, in his relation to objects, the child with autism is both fascinated and fascinating. Leo Kanner (1943) gave 'fascination with objects' as one of his six defining features of early childhood autism and described the children he had observed as having a 'skilful relationship to objects'. Persistent preoccupation with, specific attachment to and restricted, repetitive use of objects are given in the diagnostic criteria for autism of *ICD-10* (World Health Organisation, 1992) and *DCM-IV* (American Psychiatric Association, 1994). Certainly, for anyone working with children with autism, it is advisable to have great respect for and regard to a child's chosen object of interest.

The child with autism is sometimes described as having a bizarre or 'deviant' relation to objects, using them in idiosyncratic ways, different from their intended function, that are relentlessly repetitive and essentially unimaginative (Trevarthan *et al*, 1996). Moreover, favoured objects may not be ordinary toy objects but more likely hard, non-cuddly plastic toys or simple household items and tools.

The choice of a favoured object, or part of an object, is clearly sensation dominated. A child is attracted to something by its feel, appearance and the sound it makes, or by the manipulative possibilities it offers (Williams, 1992, 1996; Gerland, 1996). There is also, of course, the object's potential to shut out or keep at bay unwanted aspects of the child's world, including other people. For a child with autism, the social, cultural or symbolic meanings of the object will probably not be a factor in his fascination for it. Moreover, it is unlikely that the object will be used communicatively to develop and share social meanings.

Using people as objects is another defining feature of autism, where a person's hand, arm or body is used functionally without any sense of interpersonal contact or communication. Anybody working with autism will have had an experience of their arm used to open a door or their lap sat on as if it were a stool. You may experience eye contact that seems not to acknowledge your humanity, making you feel you are being looked through rather than at.

Donna Williams (1996) explains that, as a child, her experience of people was that they *were* objects, or part-objects with disembodied hands and mouths. In the absence of any understanding of social communication, she describes how her perception of people was based on a rich and complex set of actual sensory as well as 'felt sense' information. For her, the significant aspects of someone were located in their appearance, how they moved, how they smelled and how they made her feel, rather than in what they said or any personal connection to her.

○ The language of objects

This kind of attachment to and use of people as objects tends to be typical of a certain kind of aloof child with autism. A child who has more in the way of language and sociability may appear to relate more ordinarily to the world of objects, yet may nevertheless lack a fundamental understanding of their language and meaning.

> ⊙ **snapshot** *Leroy*
>
> *Leroy, aged eight, was working on a language activity which involved looking at pictures of ordinary scenes and answering questions. One picture showed a pair of glasses in an unusual place, on the floor of a sitting room. When the teacher asked him to say what was on the floor, he became confused and was unable to answer. He pointed correctly to the object but seemed unable to find the right word to describe it. The teacher, pointing to the glasses that were on her own face, asked, 'What are these?' Leroy replied immediately, 'Glasses', but again could not respond when his attention was directed to the picture.*

Leroy has a problem with cognition and language so that he is unable to retrieve the word for 'glasses' where the context does not give a specific visual cue. At a conceptual level, the information he holds on 'glasses' has been stored idiosyncratically, perhaps according to some sensory or perceptual feature, as opposed to any more generalised meaning.

In her vivid account of growing up as a child with autism, Gunilla Gerland gives a number of examples of the same difficulty. At one point, she describes her disappointment at being given a toy accordion for her birthday. Her understanding of 'accordion' is object-specific so that, as she writes, accordions can only be something 'beautiful, dark red and gleaming with rows of white buttons. Shiny, and with a lovely sound inside them'. When she is given a small, blue child's accordion that she cannot play, she is unable to comprehend that it is the same object (Gerland, 1996).

When knowledge of the world is stored according to an individual set of criteria, according to perceptual or sensory information say, then problems of generalisation, categorisation and shared meaning arise. Sensory-only processing of experience makes for a private 'language' that cannot be easily shared. In working with a child with autism, it is often useful to focus on semantic understanding of objects, on their properties, function and social meaning. In this way, a child's ability to think flexibly, about objects and the everyday world around him, can be developed.

○ Props, puppets and costume

Drama has a language of objects of its own, where set design, props and costume contribute to the aesthetic and overall meaning of what is being performed. In Unit 1, it was discussed how, as an art form, drama makes full use of colour, shape, texture and lighting. In drama, it is well understood that 'things' can have a life of their own. The sculptor Joseph Beuys called it the 'theatricality of objects' and argued that the dynamic of objects is not just in their appearance, but also in their use, through actions and movement with objects and arrangement.

With autism, dramatic objects can serve a further purpose. It is often the case that a child with autism prefers objects to people, showing more interest in them and feeling more comfortable communicating via them. Children with autism are attracted by the idea of puppets, masks and other talking objects and do not exhibit the same fear of them as non-autistic children. This may be because they do not perceive the same symbolic and cultural meanings, but they are drawn to them nonetheless. Of course, person-to-object communication provides an alternative to the intimacy and difficulty of person-to-person contact. Dramatic objects can provide a bridge between the two, allowing a person-to-object-to-person form of communication.

It is necessary, however, to exercise some caution when using objects. For some children, the movement, lights, noise and shininess of something can contribute to the feeling that the object is indeed alive, perhaps more alive to them than the people around. I have met children who wanted to become the object that fascinated them.

This is why it is important to 'de-role' at the end of a drama session, taking time to emphasise that the pretence has come to an end and that we have gone back to being ourselves (see Unit 9 Ending).

○ Prop boxes

A good set of props is an important preliminary to working with objects and it is possible to gradually collect items to develop a prop box. A box of everyday items is helpful when working on increasing awareness and understanding of ordinary objects, and a box of more magical things can be used with children whose imagination is more developed.

1 Everyday props

You need to consider an object in terms of:

- the shape, colour, size and texture
- what it is made of
- the function
- whether it has special properties, such as a lid, it can hold something inside, it needs power to work or it moves in an interesting way.

Choose a selection of objects that can be linked in one or more ways, having some similarities, but that are also markedly different.

Frisbee/plate (same size)	Barking dog (battery-operated)
Plastic container with lid	Power Ranger/wooden doll (same size)
Russian doll	Toothbrush (battery-operated)
Small bowl	Cleaning sponge
Wooden egg	Giant marble
Chocolate egg	Crystal
Biscuit	Small ball (orange colour)
Rectangular piece of Lego	An orange
Knife	Scissors

Most of the activities in this unit use these kinds of everyday items. However, there are a few that encourage more projective play and require objects that can be used more imaginatively. In any case, it is good practice in drama to collect interesting and thought-provoking objects with which to work that may be useful for stories, role play and improvisation.

2 Imaginative props and costume

Choose multipurpose items that will make good raw material for creating costumes, sets and props. Include beautiful, rich-looking objects, selecting carefully for colour, texture, shape or some unusual quality.

suggested items

Fabric (all colours, different textures and materials)	Coloured light
	Various hats including a crown
Cushions	Wand
Screens	Crystal ball
Tunnel	Large golden key
Parachute	Tea set
Streamers	Bags
Tubes (different sizes, soft and hard)	Phones/walkie talkies
	Pretend laptop computer
Spotlight	

In some ways, it is better to think of the group of children with whom you are working and then think of the appropriate props. Some children like reality-based play, which requires one set of props, whilst some like to be animals and others like fantasy play. A prop box could contain anything, though adaptable items such as fabric, screens and lights are basic.

Unit 5   Assessment

Area of work | Understanding & use of everyday objects & people as objects

Name of child |

Skills	Has this skill	Has demonstrated once in the group	Demonstrates regularly in the group	Has demonstrated outside the group
EVERYDAY OBJECTS	✓	DATE	DATE	DATE
1 Can name and describe according to their properties a small range of everyday objects				
2 Can name and describe according to their function and usage a small range of everyday objects				
3 Can name and describe according to their properties a wider range of everyday objects				
4 Can name and describe according to their function and usage a wider range of everyday objects				
5 Can demonstrate how an object is used, using the object				
6 Can represent through mime how an object is used				
7 Can identify one or more similarities between two objects				
8 Can identify one or more differences between two objects				
9 Can use a combination of objects to represent an everyday task				
10 Can sort objects according to a given category				
11 Can identify everyday categories for a range of familiar objects				

Skills	Has this skill	Has demonstrated once in the group	Demonstrates regularly in the group	Has demonstrated outside the group
EVERYDAY OBJECTS *(Continued)*	✓	DATE	DATE	DATE
12 Can appreciate and creatively use the sensory, sound and movement qualities of objects				
13 Can represent objects using abstract materials				
14 Can communicate via objects including puppets				
PEOPLE				
15 Notices aspects of the appearance of familiar people				
16 Can identify familiar people from a description of their appearance				
17 Can describe familiar people in terms of their appearance				
18 Can describe familiar people in terms of their role and relation to the child				
19 Can identify and create a small number of recognisable characters using costume and props				
20 Can identify and create a wider number of fictional characters using costume and props				

Notes

____

____

____

____

____

Unit 5   Aims

- To identify, describe and perform recognisable actions with a range of everyday objects

- To identify similarities and differences between two objects and sort according to given categories

- To communicate via objects and puppets

- To identify and describe familiar people according to appearance, role and relationship

- To explore abstract qualities of objects and people.

Objects and their properties

These first activities involve thinking about objects in practical, concrete terms, including such things as properties and function as well as similarities and differences between objects.

1 Definitions

This activity introduces the objects that will be used in the following two exercises.

You need

A selection of objects from your everyday items prop box.

Instruction

1 Arrange the items on a table or cloth on the floor.
2 Taking each object in turn, show the object to the group and say what it is.
3 Taking turns, ask the children to select one object and say:
   - what their object is made of
   - who usually uses it
   - where it usually is found, in the home or elsewhere.

Comment

You may need to go into the meaning of 'usually', explaining that you are thinking in 'general' terms, which may need explaining as well. You can take the activity a little further by asking children if there is an object that is usually used with their object.

2 Object mimes

Using the same selection of objects, ask the children to choose one and mime a typical action with that object.

You need

The same set of objects as for Activity 1.

Instruction

1 With the objects laid out on the table or floor, choose one and mime an action.
2 Children take turns to select an object and perform an action.
3 It is acceptable for children to select the same object to perform a different action.

Comment

Some children choose objects which can only be used to *do* the action rather than show it in a representational form, such as a ball or a Frisbee, but this is a developmental stage and should be accepted.

3 Same/different

Using the same objects, this activity focuses on similarity and difference.

You need

The same set of objects as for Activity 1.

Instruction

1 Ask the children to choose two objects and say one thing that is the same about them, or find as many similarities as they can.
2 Do this a few times with the children choosing different objects each time.
3 Go round the circle a second time, now asking the children to select two objects they have already found similar, but this time giving one or more differences.

4 What task?

In this activity, the children are required to use a set of objects together.

You need

Boxes of objects, each one containing a number of items needed to perform a particular task, for example:
- pen, paper, envelope, stamp (writing a letter)
- polish, brush, cloth (polishing shoes)
- toy, wrapping paper, sellotape, ribbon (wrapping a present).

Instruction

1 Give one box in turn to each group member and ask him to look inside it.
2 Allow time for the child to consider the contents and think of a mime.
3 The child mimes the task that the objects suggest, using the objects.
4 It is possible to include one object that is not used for that task, as a sort of joker in the pack, to see if you can catch someone out.

5 Sets

This is another way of thinking about the function and properties of ordinary everyday objects.

You need

The Sets cards (p208). If you are working with a larger group, it is possible to add more definition cards to each set.

Instruction

1 Give out the cards randomly.
2 Ask the children to find the other members of their set, specifying how many people they are looking for.
3 Some of the definition cards may apply to more than one object card, in which case children will have to discuss their set and work out who is wrongly placed.

6 Categories

Categorisation is an area with which children with autism often experience difficulty.

You need

Cards depicting ordinary objects. You can make your own using a graphics package such as *Picture This* (see Useful Contacts on p218).

Instruction

1 Tell the children that they are going to make categories of things.
2 Give each child a picture of an ordinary object.
3 Ask the children to sort themselves into two, three or more categories.
4 Ask them to decide on a label for their category and to say what is the determining criterion.

Objects and creative expression

In drama, objects can provide a powerful stimulus for work that is more creative and imaginative, and are particularly good as a basis for work with movement and sound.

7 Sensing objects

As the children become more playful, they can enjoy creative activities such as this.

You need

A selection of interesting objects from your prop box.

Instruction

1   Discuss with the children the possibility of naming objects according to a new set of criteria, for example, according to their shape, colour or the sound they make.
2   Make up words to describe the objects in the box, taking each in turn.
3   Ask the children to role play conversations where they have to ask for or talk about the object using its new name.

Extension

Tell the children that you are now not going to use words to name objects. Using one or more objects, and going round the circle, ask the children to give a movement, gesture and sound to describe the object.

8 Machine mimes

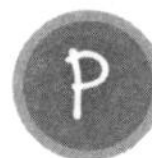 Children with autism are often fascinated by machines.

Instruction

1   Brainstorm machines that we use in our everyday lives.
2   Ask the children to choose one and develop a mime of that machine. It is a good idea to demonstrate how it is possible to be a machine, showing how you can use your body to become different machine parts.
3   Help to develop the children's ideas by asking them to choose from a list of Movement and sound words (p204), using one or two in their machine mime.
4   Ask children to show their mimes to the group.
5   Point out the possibility of using a dial that speeds up or slows down the machine.

Comment

With this activity and the next, ensure that you 'de-role' children well at the end. Machines and inventions can be particularly fascinating to a child with autism, who may want to and feel that he really has become a machine. It is important to have a good ending where you emphasise that the child is now a child again, pointing out his humanness, his fingers, hands, speaking voice and so on (for more ideas see Unit 9).

9 Inventions

Working in pairs, ask one child to invent a machine using the other child.

Instruction

1 Put the children into pairs.
2 Ask one child to invent a machine using his partner as the model.
3 He does this by giving his partner repetitive moves and some noises to make.
4 Allow the partner to practise his machine movements and sounds.
5 The inventor can press buttons to switch on the machine and the audience can say what they think is the purpose of the invention.

10 Structures

This is a highly imaginative exercise.

You need

A selection of objects, possibly ones found in the room.

Instruction

1 Clear a space and put the found objects in a pile in the centre of the room.
2 Ask the children to arrange the objects to create a structure.
3 When the structure is finished, tell the children to walk around and take a good look at it. Do they want to give it a name? What is it for? Does it do anything?
4 Dismantle the first structure and make another using the same objects.

Puppets

A puppet can be an effective resource for engaging, holding the attention of and drawing out a child with autism. Puppets are important tools for communication; the child is possibly more able to communicate with them or through them with real people. They provide a situation that is slightly indirect in terms of human communication, slightly away from faces and mouths talking, a virtual form of relating that is more comfortable. Puppets can also facilitate a graduated approach to developing communication, from puppet-to-puppet to puppet-to-person relating.

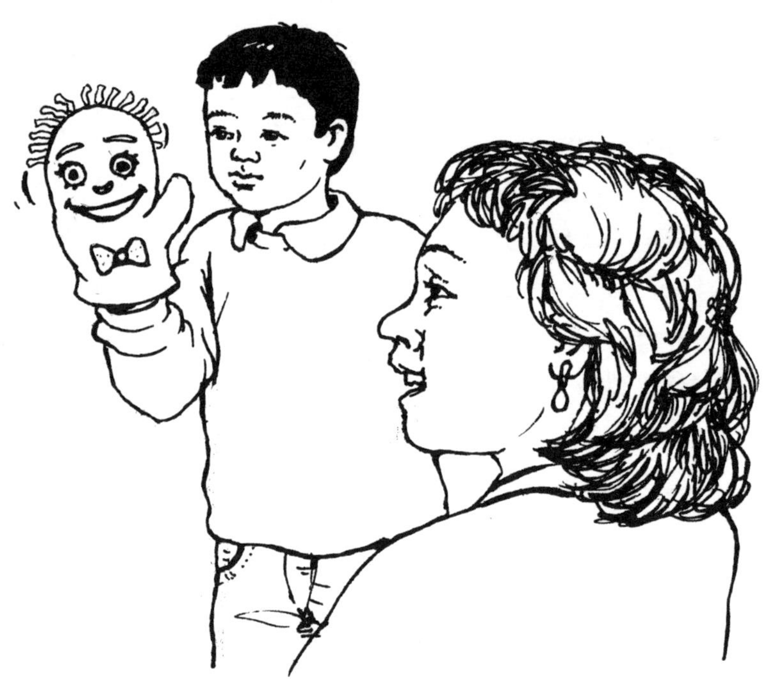

Anything can serve as a puppet and you can bring to life not just people characters but also animals and objects, making them talk and interact. Hand puppets are probably the most useful and a selection might include a man and a woman, some children, a baby, grandparent figures, a doctor, a police officer, some animals and some fairytale characters, such as a king and queen, a fairy and a witch. Children are interested in different things, some in books and stories, some in animals, some in fantasy, and you should match your puppets to the child you have in mind. For a child who is interested in cars, you could use cars as puppets choosing ones of similar size and appearance so that they create the idea of a car 'species'. Some puppets are designed specifically for communication and have moving mouths and heads. These can be particularly useful for the first activities below.

11 Talking via puppets

The idea of animating objects, having them interact and communicate with each other, is something that can be part of your general behaviour with a child and does not need to be a discrete activity within a group.

You need

A selection of hand puppets or whatever toys are to hand.

Instruction

1 Bring a box of puppets to a group session. Include actual puppets or ordinary objects that can be used in puppet-like ways.
2 Show them to the children, who should try them out, using them to converse or tell a story.
3 Model how this is done by having puppets or objects face each other and move as they talk, possibly with a put on 'character' voice. Puppets can say hello and goodbye, ask each other questions, say their names, or fight and argue.

Comment

Children's puppet play seems naturally to give rise to a lot of dramatic hitting, Punch and Judy style, and some children with autism like to do this too. At a simple level, different puppets or objects as puppets can be used to perform the same actions and say the same things.

Extension

You can introduce communication that is more humanly direct by having only one party use a puppet.

12 Acting out stories

Puppets can be used to act out stories, the children's favourites or stories of things that have actually happened.

You need

A selection of hand puppets or whatever toys are to hand.

Instruction

1 Decide on a story to be acted out. This may be a favourite story or a story about something that has actually happened to the children in the group.

2   Establish what characters there are in the story and decide which puppet
    should be which character.
3   Retell the story using the puppets.

Comment

Acting out a real-life story can serve an explanatory function where events are
played out by the puppets with an accompanying explanation of why someone
said something or reacted in the way they did. The emotional content of the
story can be pointed out in the body language of the puppet. Movement is an
important part of puppetry, and the way that a figure is moved to convey
sadness, happiness or aggression, for example, can be demonstrated and
practised.

Variation

Puppets can be used to act out and explain the meaning of common idioms such
as 'I'm all tied up now', 'He's bending over backwards for you' and 'I've got a
frog in my throat'. Use puppets to show the literal meaning and then the actual
meaning. Danielle Legler's book on idioms, *Don't Take it so Literally* (1991),
contains many more examples.

13 Talking hands

Parts of the body can be used in puppet-like ways, to say hello,
convey a piece of information or show some kind of expression.

Instruction

1   Decide on which body part you are going to use as a puppet.
2   Hands are particularly good as they can be shaped into a talking mouth,
    with flattened fingers opening and closing on the thumb, or into a walking
    figure using the first two fingers. Hands can also be moved around easily
    to suggest moving away and towards.
3   Have conversations with each other using the puppet body part.
4   Mark out expression and emotion in the way you move the body part. For
    example, moving slowly conveys sadness whilst jumping up and down
    conveys joy.
5   Use a puppet theatre, with the body hidden, as a 'stage' to move along.
    Include the use of props for the puppets.

These activities consider people as objects and are less concerned with such things as people as communicators or the roles different people play in our lives. The activities are similar to those the children have already done around actual objects and so reflect the experience that people *are* objects.

14 Whose face?

This exercise always creates lots of fun and laughter in a group and is good for building trust.

You need

A blindfold.

Instruction

1 One child is blindfolded and led to another child whose face they are allowed to feel.
2 They must give the name of the person whose face it is.
3 Alternatively, the blindfold child can feel one face and then, blindfold removed, feel all the faces of the group and say which was the original face.

Variation

If faces are too easy, try using hands or backs.

15 Smell

Lots of children express horror when this activity is suggested, but enjoy doing it anyway.

You need

A blindfold.

Instruction

1 One child is blindfolded and led to another child whose hand they smell.
2 They must name the child.
3 Alternatively, blindfold removed, the first child can smell everyone's hands and say whose was the original hand.

16 Descriptions

This activity is a good way of demonstrating that not all people have the same information in their minds.

Instruction

1 One child sits with his back to the group.
2 Quietly give another group member the name of one member of the group who they must then describe, without saying their name.
3 The child who is not looking must guess who is being described.

17 Who's different?

This activity encourages children to really look and take notice of each other.

Instruction

1 Sit in a circle and ask for a volunteer to leave the room.
2 One individual changes something about their appearance, the less obvious the better.
3 When the volunteer returns, he must guess who is different.

Comment

I often find that where a child with autism is a longstanding member of a group of peers but not necessarily one of them socially, the other children stop really *looking* at the child. It as if they know that the child is there physically but discount his presence in other ways. This activity is good to get children to notice each other again, to be reminded of all the children in the group.

18 Person definition

This activity focuses on the role of familiar people.

You need

A selection of photographs of people, ideally people the children know or who have roles with which the children are familiar.

Instruction

1 Taking each photograph in turn, ask the children to:
   - say who the person is and describe them
   - say what they do for you
   - say where they are usually found
   - describe how they make you feel.

19 Sensory portraits

Encourage children to think about familiar people in a more sensory way.

You need

Photographs of familiar people and some craft paper.

Instruction

1 Ask the children to select one photograph and attach it to the paper.
2 Add words, sentences and pictures (drawn or cut out) to describe that person.
3 Create a composite portrait using ordinary information about the person as well as sensory information and how he or she makes the child feel.
4 Ask the children to try to find ways to describe the person's smell, the sound of their voice, how they walk and move, a sensory word to describe their personality, and so on.
5 Portraits can be made into cards to give as a present to the person concerned.

20 Fantasy characters

For children who enjoy dressing up, have a session using your costume and prop box.

You need

Imaginative costume and prop box.

Instruction

1 Bring a costume box to the group.
2 The children should say what they want to be and then be helped to create that character, making a suitable outfit and finding the right props.
3 Creativity and improvisation with the materials on offer should be encouraged with the emphasis being not on accuracy but on getting the overall look right.
4 When the children are happy with their costume, take photographs of them. You can produce a 'talking photo album' (see Useful Contacts on p217) which shows the child in character and allows them to record a description of their costume and, in doing so, to say something about their character.

Me, Myself, I
Exploring aspects of the self

Introduction

Awareness of self and others is a critical area of work with autism, development here making an impact on many other areas of functioning in the child. I have often noticed how learning to name feelings and read faces can have a particularly positive effect on a child's attention, impulse control, tolerance of others and anxiety levels. However, in approaching work on the self, it does help to consider what we mean by 'me' since children with autism often have difficulty differentiating 'me' from 'you' and a poor sense of their real self.

○ Different aspects of the self

In thinking about the self, it is useful to think in terms of complex layers of self – the physical self, the social self, the feeling self – rather than a monolithic type 'me'. In some sense, 'me' is contingent upon who I am with, what I am doing and what I have experienced, rather than a fixed self that never changes or develops.

In the literature, there are different models of self, of what constitutes the self and how different aspects of the self develop. There are developmental models such as Stern's (1985) that sets out an emergent self, core self and subjective self, each becoming more sophisticated in terms of language, interaction and cognitive organisation. There are also notions of the self based on the body. Antonio Damasio (2000) outlines conscious and non-conscious aspects of self, differentiating the unconscious parts of the self that regulate bodily functions and responses from the conscious parts that form the basis of the autobiographical 'I'.

It is becoming clear that the origin of self is found in the body in relation to its environment. Developmental psychology has shown how the physical bodily experience of the infant forms the basis of self, in particular, the body's increasing capacity for self-regulation and eventually self-consciousness (Brazelton *et al*, 1974; Stern, 1985; Tronick, 1989). It is through interaction with carers and with the environment that babies develop an ability to control their inner body states as well as a sense of their own agency, or an ability to make things happen. Through this, a rudimentary sense of 'I cause therefore I am' is gained.

However, a growing sense of self also depends on the young child's capacity to differentiate himself and his actions from other people and their actions. It is a gradual sorting out process of what is 'me' and what is 'not me'. Hobson (2002) points out that the child's increasing ability to imitate and identify with other people is a part of this process and another component of self-development.

It is important, too, to consider a 'temporal self', a sense of a 'me' that existed before the present moment which can be extended into the future. Povenelli & Simon carried out research with ordinary young children, playing back video taken of them from an earlier moment in time, to show that they could recognise a present but not a delayed image of themselves. They concluded that a young child's sense of self is of a present self only and later, after the age of four, becomes a temporally extended, autobiographical self in the adult sense (Povenelli & Simon, 1998).

O Poor self-awareness in autism

Given all of this, it is unsurprising that children with autism often have poor self-awareness. It is not hard to see how autism presents a number of barriers to the development of a sense of self. Problems with sensory perception and attention, a disordered sense of the bodily self, an innate inability for interpersonal contact, poor awareness of others and absence of a theory of mind all contribute to the lack of a sense of self.

Damasio (2000) describes how a sense of self depends on a body boundary, a sense of what is in and what is outside of the self. Many children with autism pick at their skin or have an uneasy relationship with the edges of their clothes, giving the impression that this is indeed of issue. Writers with autism have described difficulty in being able to truly locate themselves in their bodies, to sense the connectedness of different parts of the body and locate feelings within it (see, for example, Williams, 1996).

Hobson describes an experiment in imitation where children with autism were able to copy an action but did not copy the *style* of the person doing the action. He argues that they missed out on an opportunity for true identification: 'Identifying with someone means recognizing the someone as a person with characteristics that one can make one's own – characteristics that come to enrich one's self' (Hobson, 2002).

Powell & Jordan (1993) have pointed out that children with autism have difficulties with 'personal episodic memory', that is, difficulty in being able to remember past events and their actions in them. They argue that the lack of an 'experiencing self' has implications for the development of an autobiographical or temporal 'I' that has a personal and social history and exists outside of the here and now.

○ True and false selves

Donna Williams has written extensively on the difficulty for people with autism of forming a real identity and true sense of self. She has described how she, like other individuals with autism, felt that 'herself' consisted of different characters, each having their own personality, forms of expression and name (Williams 1992, 1996). She points out how easy it is for people with autism to attach themselves to a false, ready-made self. The individual may choose to take on wholesale the identity of another – their mannerisms, language, emotions and even beliefs – or it may come about as the result of the rote learning and programming techniques of many interventions with autism. Whatever the cause, Williams warns against the possibility of a person with autism being split off from their true self, incapable of real experiencing and self-expression. The result may be someone who plays a role that is surface only, having no connection to an inner feeling life. I have worked with children with autism who, when asked to choose a fictional character to play, have chosen themselves.

⊙ **snapshot** *Danny*

Danny, aged 11, a boy with Aspergers, really looked forward to his weekly drama group. One week, he took part in a game called 'Party' where one child hosted a party and other children pretended to be fictional characters arriving at the party. The children chose characters they knew and liked, such as Harry Potter and Mr Fantastic, but when it came to Danny's turn he said he chose to be Danny Bates. It was pointed out to him that this was in fact himself and he became confused. When the group leader said that it was OK for him to role play himself, Danny happily rejoined the activity.

For Danny, the social self – that has a name and address, a family and goes to a school – is experienced as something quite different from the 'me' located inside. It is as if the social 'me' is experienced as a role that can be taken on or off in the same way that a child plays at being a doctor or a superhero. In fact, all of us do something like this much of the time, adopting roles to fit our immediate situation. The social anthropologist Erving Goffman argues that the construction of the self is no more than a process of taking on and performing a variety of roles, similar to dramatic roles but in actual everyday social contexts (Goffman, 1959). However, there is something less knowing and more confused in Danny's taking on of himself as a role, and it is important in drama with children with autism to be clear that '*this* is real and *this* is pretend'.

It will be apparent how rich a resource drama is when thinking about the self. The very fact that drama provides an opportunity for role play whilst focusing on the body and on the individual in different situations means that there is great scope for exploring the different aspects of 'me'.

O Role in drama

In drama, the notion of role reflects to some degree the sociological idea of 'function' within, for example, the family, group or society in general. It would differ from the idea of character in the sense that the latter concerns a more fully realised dramatic persona. Examples of role would be brother, friend, policeman or leader. Jennings (1987) defines role as a pattern of behaviour: actions carried out sufficiently often for a pattern to emerge. She points out that roles are generally relational since actions usually relate to something or someone. Roles are often presented in terms of their dyadic or oppositional partner, such as brother and sister, friend and enemy, policeman and crook, leader and followers. In order for a role to appear convincing in drama, it is necessary for the role-taker to have a number of prerequisite skills which include:

- the ability to carry out pretend actions
- the ability to imagine what the subject of the role might say or feel
- the ability to imagine how the subject of the role might respond to something or someone.

Role play typically involves improvisation, imagined dialogues and enactment of scenes, all of which would call on the above. Drama workshop activities may also explore role through a variety of methods such as role reversing and doubling, where the thoughts of someone in role are imagined and spoken aloud by members of the group.

O Development of role play in young children

These skills clearly reflect the ordinary development of dramatic role play in young children. First (1994) outlines three stages of development of dramatic play, beginning with the simple role reversal of I ⇔ you, where the self represented in the play is the child's own self and the 'you' a very familiar other, such as the mother. From here, the child develops the capacity for a greater number of roles, usually in dyadic relation – doctor/patient, mother/baby, big one/little one – and all within close experience. The final stage is characterised by the child being able to assume a multiplicity of roles and role reversals, still in dyadic relation. First (1994) concludes that 'the capacity to assume pretend roles depends on the ability to put oneself in another's place'.

Clearly, autistic difficulty with theory of mind is at issue here. Theory of mind means being able to suspend belief in the here and now, to adopt false beliefs and pretend stances, to act upon 'as if' and put oneself into the shoes of another. Children with autism lack a theory of mind and so are prevented from developing this level of sophistication in play. The activities that follow will suggest ways of structuring drama that allow a child to access role play and use it to adopt and explore the familiar roles of everyday life.

○ The activities

The activities in this unit explore each aspect of the self separately. Children are encouraged to share personal facts and to consider themselves in terms of what they have achieved in their life. The focus will then turn to the emotional self, the 'feeling me', and to what our experiences mean in terms of how they make us feel. The roles that we typically play will then be explored. Role will be looked at in terms of the actions we perform and things we say in our different social settings, how they relate to the people in our lives as well as to our general sense of self. Finally, there will be some suggestions for working on the roles that children adopt in the drama group itself and how to work with shifting those in which they feel stuck.

Unit 6   Assessment

Area of work | Awareness of self & others

Name of child |

Skills	Has this skill	Has demonstrated once in the group	Demonstrates regularly in the group	Has demonstrated outside the group
PERSONAL DETAILS	✓	DATE	DATE	DATE
1 Can share personal facts				
2 Can provide facts about other people who are familiar				
3 Can relate significant life events				
4 Can share own achievements				
5 Can identify significant people in own life				
EMOTIONS				
6 Can recognise and show happiness and sadness using facial expression and body posture				
7 Can provide situations of happiness and sadness, with reasons				
8 Can recognise and show anger and fear using facial expression and body posture				
9 Can provide situations of anger and fear, with reasons				
10 Can name, recognise and show a variety of emotions using facial expression and body posture				

Unit 6   Assessment *(Continued)*

Skills	Has this skill	Has demonstrated once in the group	Demonstrates regularly in the group	Has demonstrated outside the group
EMOTIONS *(Continued)*	✓	DATE	DATE	DATE
11 Can provide situations, with reasons, for a variety of emotions				
12 Can recall and discuss a recent incident in terms of its emotional content				
13 Shows understanding of different intensities of emotion				
14 Can comment on the quality of a feeling				
15 Can explain likes and dislikes				
ROLE				
16 Can name common social roles				
17 Can identify own social roles, providing one or more details				
18 Can identify familiar combinations of roles				
19 Can identify roles of individuals in the group				
20 Can take on a new role within the group				

Notes

____

____

____

____

Unit 6   Aims

◎ To develop self-awareness including of own physical attributes, personality, family and personal history

◎ To be able to recognise, name and communicate own feelings and compare them with other people's feelings

◎ To link emotion to real-life events

◎ To improve self-esteem.

Unit 6   Activities

Group interaction and trust

With group work, an essential preliminary to exploring aspects of the self is first establishing a sense of safety, trust and to some extent belonging within the group. Personal details and histories, and exploring feelings and personality, are inevitably sensitive issues. It is important to remember too that greater self-awareness comes through interpersonal contact and an awareness of others.

The child with autism often feels himself to be an outsider to his group of peers. The possibility of this will have been minimised to some extent in the putting together and setting up of the group. However, it is often the case that the child does not have any real link or bond to his peers and does not feel or is not felt to be part of his peer group. What follows are group 'gelling' exercises and activities to promote trust without requiring too much in the way of physical contact, a typical component of this kind of work. There is also some element of doing something with personal details, giving a taste of what follows in the rest of the programme.

1 Anyone who

All children, of almost any age, love this game. It is a simple but effective way of pointing out what is shared within the group and is good as a standard opener.

Instruction

1 The group sit on chairs in a circle with only enough chairs for those sitting down.
2 One person stands in the middle of the circle and says, *'Anyone who…'*, finishing the sentence with some detail of themselves such as the colour of their hair, the first letter of their name, if they have a brother. They might say, *'Anyone who is wearing black shoes'*, *'Anyone who has a cat'*, *'Anyone whose favourite film is* Lord of the Rings'.
3 It is important to remember that the statement must be true for the child who is saying it, since children often forget this.
4 People for whom this statement is also correct, that is, those group members who are wearing black shoes and so on, must then swap seats.
5 The object of the game is for the person in the middle to sit on a chair.
6 The person who is left standing begins the game again, starting with a new *'Anyone who…'*.

2 Group juggle

It is a good idea to do the juggle at the beginning of sessions, asking children to choose each time a different child to catch the ball.

You need

Two or three balls.

Instruction

1 Group members stand higgledy-piggledy around the space.
2 The leader throws a ball to one person who must then throw it to a different person, who throws it to another and so on until it comes back to the leader.
3 Ask the children to remember to whom they threw the ball, thereby establishing a 'route'.
4 Once the route of the ball has been established begin to juggle by again throwing in the ball, with group members throwing it to their chosen person.
5 Allow the ball to go round the group a few times before introducing another ball and then, possibly, another.
6 As the balls are juggled, a group rhythm should be set up and a bond established between the people who are passing it to one another.

Comment

Soft foam balls and koosh balls are easy to catch and throw and could be used.

Me, the facts

A good place to start work about ourselves is to focus on the 'neutral' territory of sharing straightforward personal details, such as our address, when we were born and who is in our family. This means that work on the self begins with activities that focus on our strengths and talents. Many children with autism worry about what they are not good at and feel that they have many shortcomings, so it is a good idea to give self-esteem a boost right from the start.

3 Numbers and letters

This is a Chris Johnston game that is good to use with a child who is fascinated by numbers and letters (Johnston, 1998).

Instruction

1 Put the children into pairs or threes.
2 Ask them to make a shape, a number or a letter.
3 Link the numbers and letters to personal details of group members, such as birthday dates, height, age or how many times they have achieved something.

Variation

If the activity is a challenging one for the focus child, it is possible to do the activity in the middle of the circle, one small group at a time, and so provide support. However, it is also possible to do it as a whole group activity by asking the children to move around the space and then calling out the shape, number or letter. The children must quickly find a partner and act on the instruction.

4 Lining up

A fun way of sharing pieces of personal information in a group.

You need

A line marked out on the floor with masking tape, long enough to accommodate the whole group.

Instruction

1   Tell the children that the object of the game is to form a line but they must establish who is first, second, third and so on according to some given criteria.
2   Base the criteria on some personal detail: the months of the year in which your birthday falls, age, height, house number.
3   You need to indicate which end of the line is the beginning, that is, January, the youngest, the shortest, the lowest number.
4   The group must sort themselves out along the line.
5   When they are in their order, check they have got it right by individuals calling out their age, height or whatever.

Extension

Repeat the activity but this time tell the group they must sort themselves out without saying anything. They can use gesture, pointing, facial expression and signs, but not words to work out who stands where. It is interesting at this point to see how the children negotiate the task and who the leaders are.

5 Child poem

Harnessing the group's collective experience of the child, this activity focuses solely on the child's strengths and can provide a powerfully positive experience.

You need

Large sheets of different coloured paper and a marker pen.

Instruction

1   Have the children sit in a circle and say that each child will have a turn at being the focus of the group.
2   Ask for a volunteer and write his name at the top of the paper.
3   Invite the group to brainstorm all the things that he is good at doing, saying only positive things.
4   Write down all the children's ideas. If a child's comment is not that positive, such as *'Talks a lot'*, ask them to rephrase it or do not write it down.
5   It is possible to pass on being the focus child, but not on providing comments.
6   Wait for ideas until the paper is completely full.

7 When all the children have had a turn at being the focus child, using a different coloured paper for each, say that you will type them up and give them back later.

8 In writing out a child's positive comments, try to introduce a poetic element so that what was a list becomes a kind of poem. You might need to group some of the statements or rephrase them a little, and add 'You're' every so often.

9 Write the child's name at the top as a title and return it as if you are giving a special gift.

Comment

I find that children make wonderful comments about other children that are kind, thoughtful, straightforward and authentic, giving ideas which an adult would never think of. I have often seen children glow with pride and self-esteem as they listen to all these good things. Children often make comments such as *'Nice to be with'*, *'Good to talk to'*, *'A good friend'*, which are just the sorts of thing a child with autism needs to hear.

⊙ child poem for a girl

Megan

You think you are good at dancing.
Your friends think you are
Good at maths and science
Good at writing
Good at painting and drawing –
You're a creative person
And write nice poems.
You're a fast reader
You're good at using a calculator.
You're kind
You're quiet
You're a good friend
You've got a good imagination
You're good at playing – you don't mind who you play with
You're never in trouble – you'll always do as you are told
You keep your promises
You've got a good character.

Tom

You think you're good on Playstation.
Your friends think you are
Good at music especially on the recorder
Good at maths
Good at running
And you can swim.
You're good at collecting Yu-Gi-Oh cards
And good at remembering things.
You're funny – you've got a good sense of humour
You cheer people up
You're good with small children
You're fun to play with
You're good at acting out scenes from films.
You help with your baby brother
You find good hiding places
You think up good spells.

6 Social map

Children explore visually the social relationships in their lives.

You need

Paper and pen for each child.

Instruction

1 Instruct individuals to draw a 'map' showing their social network. They should write 'Me' in a circle in the centre and then draw lines going out to join up with significant people in their life.

2 Consideration should be given to how far and where to locate the other people. Are they 'close' socially, or not that close? Are they close in terms of distance, but not that close in terms of relationship? (See Figure 6.1)

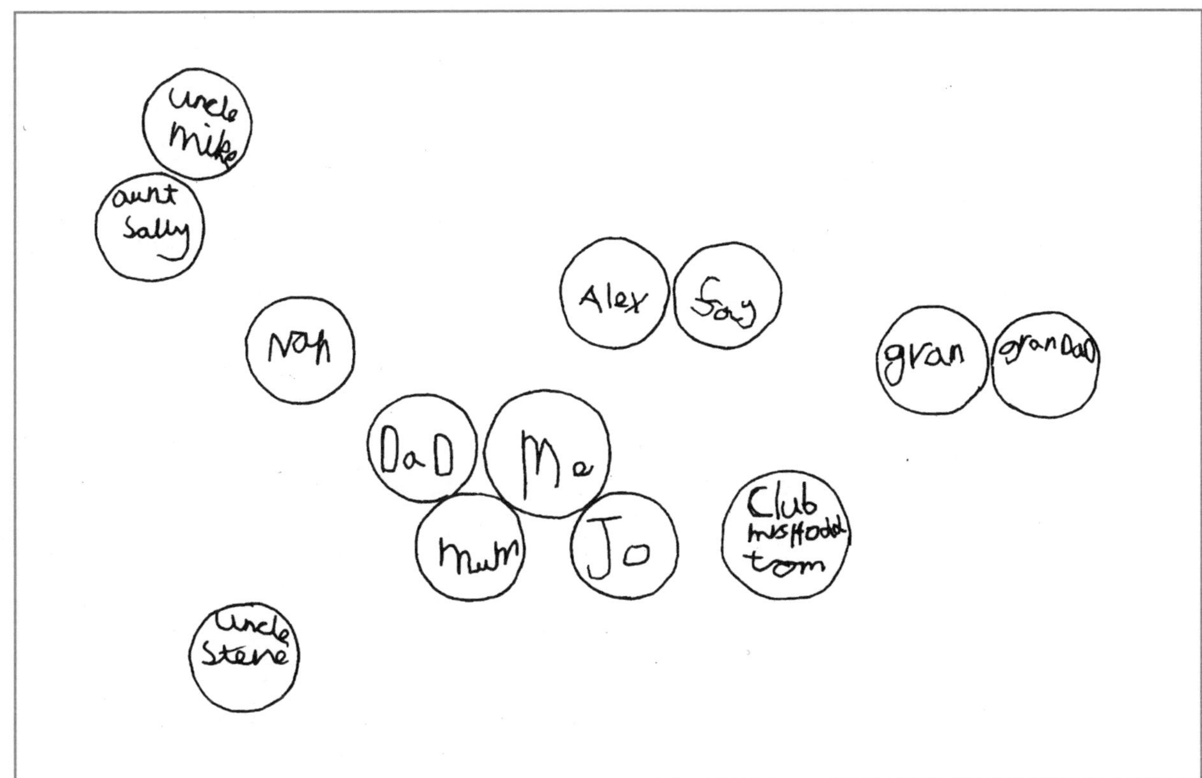

Figure 6.1 Example of a social map

Comment

A child's social map may have very little life in it so to speak, containing few significant people, or it may not truly reflect the actual circumstances of his life. This may be an indication of what the child believes to be true. However, it is possible to work on this by asking other people in the child's life – teacher, parent, another child in the class – to create their social map for that child. This can act as a point of comparison to the child's own map and give an alternative view of their social life.

Feeling me

Working with feelings is rarely easy or straightforward. For children with autism, poor self-awareness, poor body awareness and theory of mind difficulties can add to the task. Temple Grandin (Grandin & Johnson, 2005) argues that people with autism actually function differently in terms of feeling from non-autistic people, having simpler, more straightforward emotions which are seldom mixed. However, working on feelings is crucial and can have an impact on the development of the whole self. I have worked with children whose capacity for self-regulation has dramatically improved after work has been done on recognising, naming and expressing their own and other people's emotions.

⊙ snapshot *Joe*

Joe, aged five, displayed very difficult behaviours in the classroom setting. These included hitting and scratching other children, attacking his support worker, throwing himself onto the carpet and going under furniture. It was clear that, whilst he was interested in the other children and keen to be part of the group, the whole environmental experience of school was difficult for him. Much work had been done in terms of cognitive behavioural support, but his support worker had also done some work on naming and recognising feelings, putting up an emotions wall to show expressions of simple emotions. An occasion arose where Joe lashed out at another child and then hid under a table. His support worker left him for a while and then, going to the table, quietly asked him, 'Do you feel sad?' Joe immediately came out from under the table and sought a hug, which he received. His acting out behaviour, which usually escalated, had suddenly disappeared.

Damasio (2000) makes a useful distinction between emotions and feelings. He points out that 'emotion' involves the outward bodily response to an internal or external stimulus and is usually public and observable. 'Feeling', on the other hand, involves the inward, private mental experience of that emotion. He also makes distinctions between different categories of emotion, including the six basic emotions of fear, anger, sadness, disgust, surprise and happiness, and social emotions such as embarrassment, jealousy and pride. There are also background emotions which are sustained over a period of time and may very well be unconscious. Examples of these are a sense of well-being, contentment, tension, edginess and relaxation.

When exploring this aspect of the self, it is a good idea to consider whether you are working on an emotion, the outward physical display, or the experience of that emotion for the individual, the feeling. It is also helpful to tackle one emotion at a time. Most children, including many children with autism, seem early on to recognise happiness and sadness in others. However, they may attribute every good emotional display to 'happiness' and every negative or neutral display to 'sadness'. It can be hard to encourage a deeper understanding of basic emotions, but tackling them individually does help. Try to separate out different aspects of the subject and work on each in turn:

- recognising emotions, knowing their name and how they appear
- situations that give rise to particular emotions
- different intensities of feeling
- the quality or 'feel' of a feeling.

7 Body awareness

This activity is a warm-up for working on feelings by drawing the child's attention to different parts of his body and considering 'pleasant' and 'unpleasant' feelings.

Instruction

1 Ask the group to get comfortable and then concentrate on what you are going to say. They can have their eyes open or closed, though closed does help more with concentration.
2 Tell the children to become aware of different parts of themselves, the toes, knees, back and so on, giving them a little time to focus on each.
3 You can be specific, saying which toe, which knee, which finger or what part of the head. You can also suggest feeling the clothing or objects that touch a part of the body: the trouser on your leg, the collar round your neck, the earring in your ear.

Variation

It is possible to give an exaggerated experience of the body, and thus aid awareness, by asking the child to touch objects with unusual textures. Examples would be ice, fur, sandpaper, ribbon, an egg. Ask the children to consider which are 'nice' and 'not nice' to touch. Point out that when we touch something pleasant our body is 'open' to the experience, but when it encounters something unpleasant it naturally withdraws.

8 Emotions wall

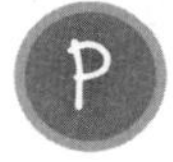 These next two activities focus on the naming and recognition of basic emotions.

You need

Stories, pictures and photographs depicting target emotions (see Emotions pictures, p209). Good books to use with younger children are to be found in Useful Contacts at the end of this book.

Instruction

1 Using your resources and taking the basic emotions in turn, spend some time exploring what each looks like and typical events that give rise to it. Consider:
   - the physical aspects of an emotion, eg that happiness means a smiling face, bright eyes and an open face and body
   - alternative words for the emotion
   - whether it is a 'nice' or 'not nice' feeling
   - whether it is a short feeling, over with quickly, or whether it tends to go on for a long time.
2 Start to create an emotions wall by mapping out areas of feelings and adding your pictures to the appropriate section.
3 Add more pictures, words and photos to create a collage of that feeling on the wall. Look out for the children themselves showing some of these emotions and include photographs of them with a brief explanation of what was happening at the time.
4 It is worth pointing out that most of the time we are in a balanced state of feeling, or neutral state, and you might want to make space for this on your wall too.

Comment

Whatever the structure, try to make the wall highly visual, using pictures, photographs, colour, lettering and patterns, trying to convey some quality of that feeling in the display.

Extension

Depending on the needs of the child, the wall can simply be a display of faces showing the basic facial expressions which are then labelled (see Figure 6.2). However, if the child is more able, you can structure your emotions wall in some way. A useful way of dividing emotions is into those that give rise to comfortable and uncomfortable feelings. Alternatively, try to group similar feelings together and have a perimeter area for longer-term background emotions and feelings as well (see Figure 6.3).

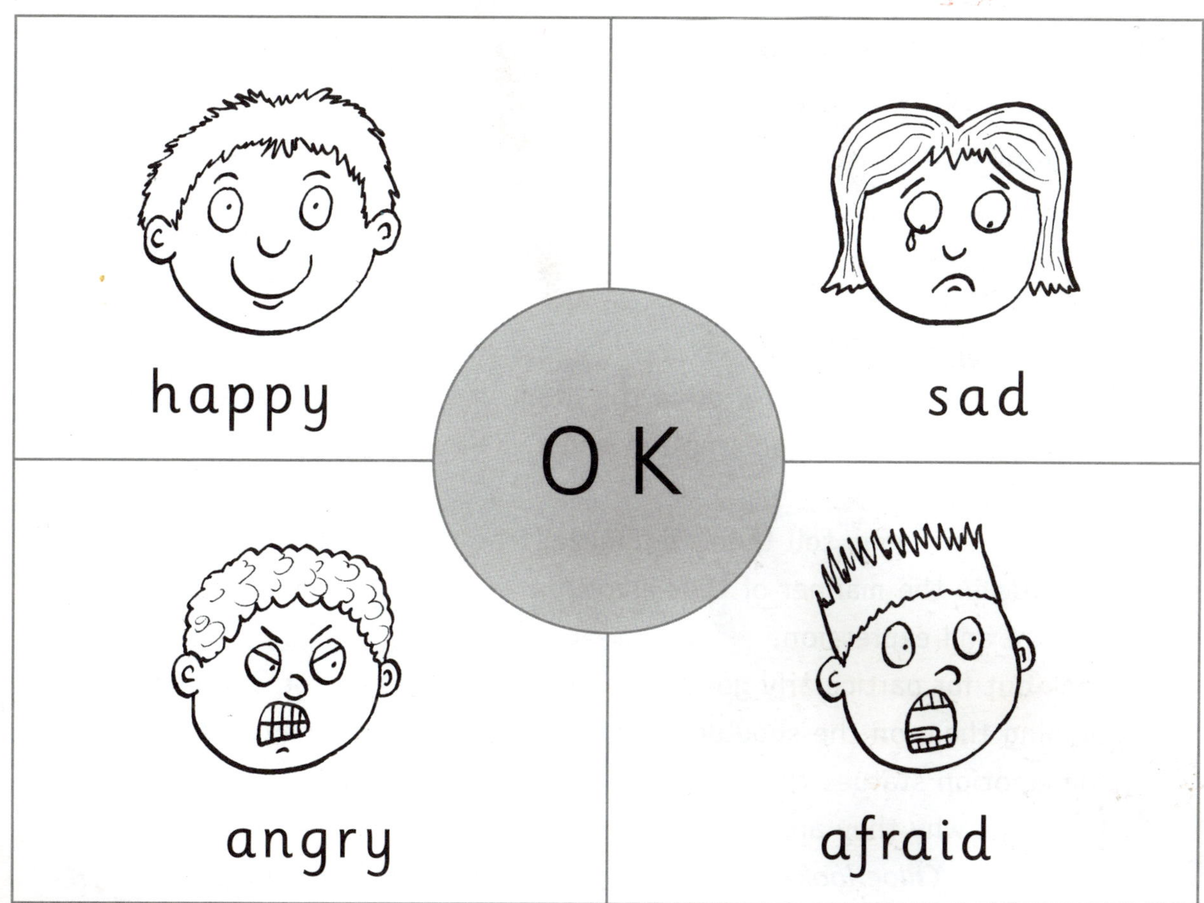

Figure 6.2 Simple emotions wall showing the four basic feelings and neutral state

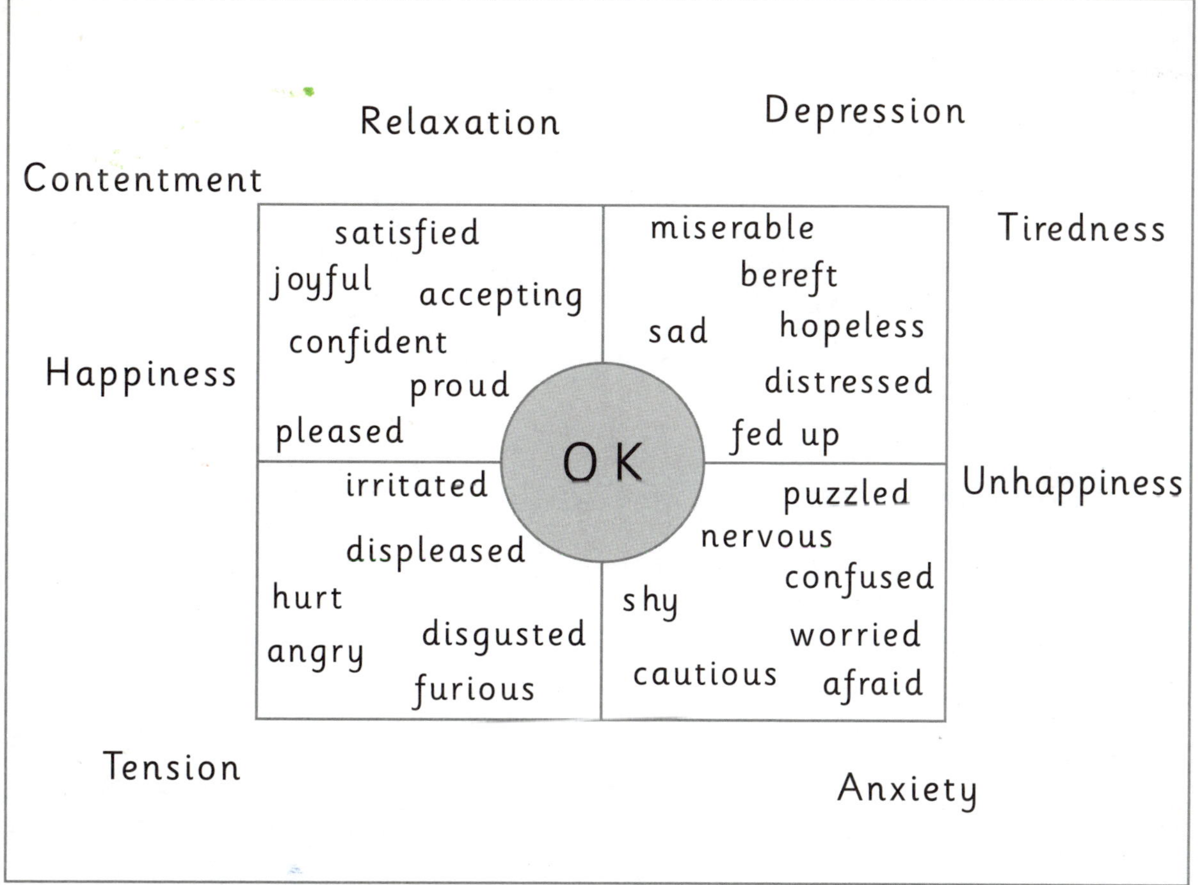

Figure 6.3 Emotions wall showing more complex emotions and background feelings

9 Emotion statues

This activity gives children the opportunity to look closely at emotional expression in others and to try out facial expressions for themselves.

Instruction

1 Brainstorm different emotions.
2 Ask the children to walk around the room, maintaining a steady pace.
3 As they walk, call out an emotion and tell them to think about what it looks like.
4 After a short time, tell them to 'Freeze!' The children should stand still like a statue in the manner of that emotion, trying to convey it through their posture and expression.
5 Look out for particularly good examples and release some children by tapping them on the shoulder and telling them to walk around and look at the emotion statues that remain.
6 Point out why they are successful, for example: *'Joe looks happy because he is smiling'*, *'Chloe looks sad because she is crying'*, *'Tina is frightened and she is hiding her face so she can't see.'*
7 Use a mirror to show the child how he is successfully expressing an emotion.

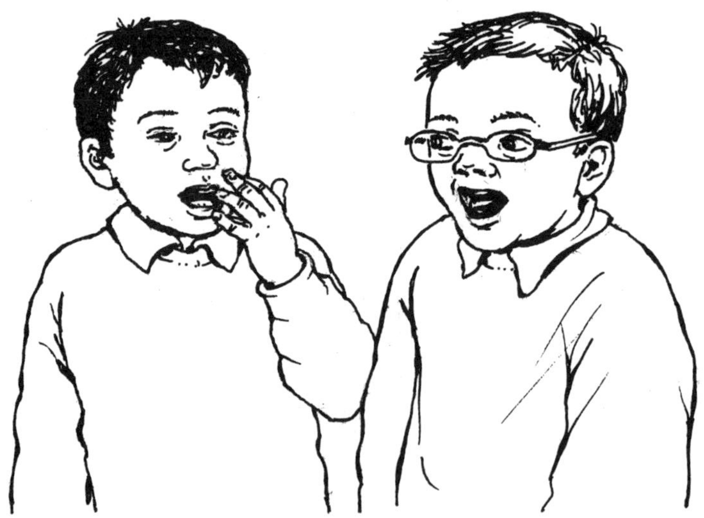

Variation

With the children in pairs facing each other, one as the leader and one the mirror image, ask them to perform emotion mirrors. The lead child expresses different emotions in his body, making slow and steady movements. The mirror image tries to reflect these as precisely as possible so that the leader can 'see' his emotions as he displays them.

10 Remembering yesterday

This activity, together with the two that follow, concentrate on the situational context of ordinary, everyday emotions.

Instruction

1 Ask the children to sit quietly, relax and concentrate.
2 Tell them to think about their bodies and then try to remember what they did that morning.
3 Ask questions to prompt memory: What time did they wake up? Did they get up straight away or go back to sleep? What was the first thing they did when they got out of bed? What did they eat for breakfast?
4 They should try to go through what they did, reliving the experience in their bodies, thinking about their bodily sensations as they recall their actions.
5 When the morning has been remembered, ask the children to go back further in time, to the previous evening, and repeat the exercise.

11 Focusing

Eugene Gendlin (1978) devised a method of focusing which can be used to explore a single event by combining thought, feeling and body sensation. For individuals with autism, who have difficulty recalling events as they happen to them, this exercise helps to make that link. It can powerfully evoke recent events and stimulate an account and discussion of what has happened.

Instruction

1 Children need to choose a recent and significant event, perhaps one from the previous exercise.
2 They should find a space on a chair or on the floor where they are comfortable.
3 When everyone is settled, begin the focusing exercise using the following questions:
   ◉ Think about your event, but don't go into it.
   ◉ What do you sense in your body when you think of what happened? Give your attention to that body sensation.
   ◉ Try to sense all the feeling involved.
   ◉ What is the quality of the felt sense – what one word, phrase or image comes into mind?
   ◉ In your mind, go back and forth between the felt sense and the words or image. Are they a right match?

⊙ If the felt sense changes, follow it with your attention.

⊙ When the felt sense and the words or image match, this is focusing.

4 Ask the group to make a circle and share their experience of the focusing exercise.

5 Ask individuals what sensations they felt and what is their word, phrase or image.

6 Encourage individuals to consider the event in the light of what they have learned from the focusing exercise.

7 Ask them if, by finding a word, phrase or image, they have learned something new about what happened.

Comment

The work can be done individually, for a child who needs support to focus, or in a group.

12 Feeling gauge

It is helpful to point out the fact that a feeling can be experienced at different levels of intensity, from pleasure to joy or from nervousness to fear.

You need

A gauge drawn out on a piece of card and divided it into six equal parts, marked 0–5. Attach some kind of indicator, such as a moving arrow or push-along window.

Instruction

1 Ask the children to brainstorm words and phrases to describe the intensity of feelings, for example, 'a bit', 'quite', 'very', 'really', 'totally'.

2 Decide where each should go on the gauge and write them in.

3 Use the gauge to measure the intensity of feeling of an incident recalled from one of the last two exercises.

Extension

It is possible to use the gauge to chart the intensity of one particular feeling. Taking happiness, for example, ask the group to think of a word to describe a little bit of happiness, quite a bit of happiness, total happiness, and so on. Use these to make a 'Happiness Gauge'.

13 Shopping for feelings

The last two activities in this section on feelings focus on the 'quality' of feelings, trying to give some sense of what a feeling feels like.

You need

A variety of containers – bottles, jars, boxes, packages – of different shapes and sizes and with the labels removed or covered. Some blank sticky labels.

Instruction

1 Thinking about the quality of the feelings discussed so far, ask the group to decide which container should be used for which feeling.
2 Ask the children to give their reasons. Anger, for example, might need to be kept in a jar with a good screw-on lid so that it cannot get out easily, whilst happiness might be stored in the prettiest container.
3 Instruct the children to make labels for the containers and decide on a price, working out what each feeling is worth.
4 Arrange the containers on shelves and role play shopping for feelings. One child is given an event for which he needs some feelings, for example, for his birthday or for when he is told off by his teacher. He should then ask another child, as the shopkeeper, to provide the appropriate feelings.

14 Colour, shape, sound

This is a creative activity that may not be suitable for some children with autism, though some will really enjoy it.

Instruction

1 In a round, ask the children to take turns to complete the sentence, *'If happiness were a colour it would be...'*
2 Use the basic emotions, or whatever feelings you are working on, and try a variety of categories, such as colour, shape and sound.
3 When the children come up with different ideas for the same feeling, point out that our experience of feelings is highly personal.

Variation

Do the same activity to encourage the expression of feeling in language. Ask the group to begin with *'If anger were a word it would be...'*, covering different emotions, and then move on to, *'If it were a phrase or sentence it would be...'*.

This last activity is moving the children into the realm of improvisation and their ideas could be used for a scene sculpt. Ask the children to create a sculpt of two people experiencing a particular emotion. Once they have established the sculpt – their position in relation to each other and the activity they are engaged in – ask them to freeze but keep in mind their sentence attached to that emotion. You can then touch a child lightly on the shoulder to prompt them to speak their line and so bring the scene to life.

Finally, the activities in this section on role will help to develop an awareness of the 'social self', particularly as it relates to significant others. As a preliminary to the work, it is helpful to discuss the meaning of the word 'role', pointing out that one person can have many different roles depending on what they are doing and whom they are with.

15 The empty chair

This activity introduces work on role by asking the children to think about what roles they play in life.

You need

A pen, a large sheet of paper and an extra chair.

Instruction

1 Brainstorm all the different roles we have.
2 Write out the children's ideas on a large sheet of paper.
3 Ask the children to identify which roles they have played in the last week, taking ideas from the brainstorm or thinking of their own.
4 Ask the children to think of one of their roles and think of an action, movement or gesture that goes with it.
5 Go round the circle asking children to show their movement.
6 Ask the children to think of or write down a sentence that goes with that role, something they typically say when they are carrying out that role.
7 Set out an empty chair, with the group facing it as the audience.
8 Ask the children to take it in turns to sit in the empty chair, or stand by it, to perform their movement and say their line.
9 Repeat the exercise, asking the children to choose another of their roles.

16 Role + action

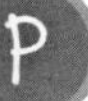

Sue Jennings (1987) gives an alternative way of identifying the roles we play in life, focusing on the actions implicit in a role.

You need

Role cards (p210).

Instruction

1 Set out the role cards and instruct the children to choose two or three that apply to them.

2   Ask them to write a sentence about each role starting *'I am the sort of person who...'* and completing them with the actions they usually perform in this role. Examples would be *'plays with my friends'*, *'helps my mum at home'*, *'worries about school'.*

3   Ask the children to share with the group what are the roles they most regularly play.

Extension

Roles can be explored further by adding an adverb to describe how they carry out their various roles, for example, 'plays frantically', 'listens distractedly'. Movement and sentences can again be created to bring these roles to life.

17 Paired roles

Using some of the ideas generated in the previous exercises, this activity looks at how we play social roles in relation to other people.

Instruction

1   Explain that the roles we have in life are usually in relation to another person and their role.

2   Children should work out who in the group has a compatible role. If they talk a lot, for example, they may be compatible with someone who listens, but not compatible with someone who likes to spend time by themselves or who is fed up with listening.

3   In pairs, invite the children to sit in two empty chairs and perform their roles together using the movements and sentences generated in the previous exercise.

4   Give some preparation time to work out what to say and do and how to put the two roles together.

Extension

Perform role plays of roles that are non-compatible, discussing the problems that ensue. For example, a talker combined with someone who does not listen may result in frustration and anger.

Exploring roles in the group

It is often the case that individuals adopt particular roles when put into a group situation. Here are a selection of activities to explore the roles present in the group.

1 Explain how we often take on specific roles within a group situation.
2 Give examples of typical group roles: listener, talker, helper, partner, thinker, leader, follower, team member, individual. The group may be able to work these out for themselves.
3 Choose from amongst the following activities to explore some of these roles more deeply, thinking which would be particularly relevant to *this* group.

18 Blind walk (helping and trust)

Blindfold one person and ask another to be a helper, guiding him around an obstacle course. Discuss the essential role of a helper, emphasising the importance of thinking about the needs of the other person and of keeping them safe. Think about how that could be done in this exercise, for example, by talking to the blindfolded person, reassuring them and explaining where they are going. Give different children the opportunity to be a helper.

19 Who's the leader? (leading and following)

Ask for a volunteer to leave the room. Sitting in a circle, decide on one person to be 'leader'. This means that everyone must sit in the same way as the leader and copy any pose or movement he makes. Advise the leader to make only small, subtle movements, giving some examples. Bring the volunteer back into the room and ask them to stand in the circle. After watching the group move, the volunteer must work out who is the leader. Every child should have the opportunity of being the leader.

20 Floating (team spirit)

Children sit in chairs set out higgledy-piggledy, with one empty chair. One person is 'It' and must walk around the space trying to sit down. The group needs to work together to prevent this by moving from chair to chair, ensuring he or she cannot sit down. It is important that the person who is 'It' maintains a steady walking pace, since it is tempting to speed up and rush to an empty chair.

Storytelling
Recalling events/making meaning

Introduction

At its simplest level, a story is a sequence of events involving one or more characters in a setting, linked in some way that serves to create an overall meaning. A story differs from a narrative in that it has more about it in the way of aesthetic and design, the latter being an everyday form of relating that occurs in ordinary conversations (Cattanach, 1997). A story has a 'format', a recognisable structure for the account with which the listener may be familiar. The meaning of the story, moreover, is contained in more than the retelling of events. Storyline and character will probably contribute and may signify certain universally recognisable themes, qualities, motivations and intentions. In stories, plot conflicts tend to move towards resolution whilst a character's role often signifies their innate qualities, choices and actions (hero = strong, brave and good).

Children with autism often have difficulty telling stories, both real and imagined. They may find it hard to give an account of what has happened to them in ordinary life, not having experienced events in the same way as someone who does not have autism. They may also have difficulty in listening to stories and understanding the details. The actions of characters in a story may not be understood, and the affective content and overall gist not fully appreciated. Stories are usually concerned with a character's inner motives and drives and, given theory of mind difficulty, this can be an obstacle to real understanding.

○ Problems with narrative

In Bruner & Feldman's (1993) interesting study on language use and autism, they found that the real problem with language and interaction is the limited ability to generate narratives. Their research shows that people with autism will give an account of something that has happened which is shorter, more descriptive or report-like in substance and contains fewer links between action and purpose than that given by a non-autistic person. It will be more a list of things that happened rather than a reconstruction of events composed in such a way as to create some overall perceived meaning.

Bruner & Feldman point out how pervasive a narrative-type structure is to ordinary children's cognition and communication at all stages of development. Children as young as two and three years of age will make up stories to help them understand ordinary things that have happened, posing puzzles about events and resolving them with problem-solving narratives. In this way, they develop their understanding by building 'canonical representations of how the world of people-and-things works and should work' (Bruner & Feldman, 1993). The young child's ability to generate narratives may be linked to his early experiences of interaction with a carer, the format of which contains a narrative drive: the interaction begins, there is a shared action which has meaning, the interaction is brought to an end in some way.

For older children, their use of language is narrative based with an important component of ordinary discourse being a 'topic-comment' structure, the child taking as a topic what has just been said and using it as a basis for their subsequent comment. Their language too has a high content of narrative-drive words, such as *but, so, because, then, before* and *later,* as well as words to describe people's intentional states and reasons for doing things (Bruner & Feldman, 1993).

By contrast, the typical language use of a child with autism contains few or none of these features. Significantly, Bruner & Feldman found that children with autism do not use a topic-comment structure, seldom picking up on what has been said and not knowing how to make a new comment on it. They use fewer pragmatic words in retelling stories and their accounts have less content about why, where and how something happened. In fact, it is speculative whether children with autism have a canon of narrative formats in mind, not having built one up from early experiences of interaction in the same way as non-autistic children.

O Autistic perception

However, problems with narrative relate not only to the disordered development of language in a child with autism but also to his perceptual experience of the world. As Jordan & Powell (1995) have pointed out, people with autism cannot reflect on experience because they do not properly have a sense of themselves having that experience in the first place. An individual experiences things non-subjectively so that he does not have a sense of something happening *to him*. There is a gap between the event and the feelings associated with that event, which in turn leads to problems with being able to properly process and recall what has happened. Our cues to memory are emotional and the absence of an experiencing self means there is no cue to remembering something that has happened, though the memory of the events might be intact and available for recall if cued externally.

Added to this are autistic difficulties with attention so that what is seen is observed in great visual detail but with little understanding of any personal and social content. In such circumstances it is difficult to perceive meaning in events or have an overall idea of what is going on. Donna Williams (1996) describes it as difficulty in attention, perception and systems integration and defines it as a general problem of 'connectedness'.

○ A storytelling curriculum

The learning needs around stories for a child with autism thus involve learning to listen to and recall, to understand and retell stories. The teaching challenge is to provide structures for both experiencing and retelling stories. However, what is really at issue is developing a mental capacity to make meaningful connections between things, to have a sense of what is going on, to be able to think about it and communicate it.

The activities that follow aim to gradually build up the skills needed to do this, beginning with the ability to make realistic and sensible links between two, three or more things in everyday contexts. Different ways of telling stories are given, from simple to more complex, which will allow the child to have experience of and practice in using a range of storytelling formats. Stories are also broken down into their component parts, of characters, setting and sequence of events, as a way of attending to the important details of what is happening and to aid the retelling of stories. Props are used as objects of reference to cue the memory of important details and also for the purposes of retelling.

It is recommended that the stories used include events from the students' own lives, whether everyday occurrences or one-off incidents. However, there is mileage in using published stories as well, particularly well-known stories with clear and recurring structures and themes, such as fairy tales and folktales. It can also be useful to use picture books for younger children with older children, who tend to like the strong visual element and may be more able to identify with the social and emotional content.

Finally, difficulties in the area of storytelling can have knock-on effects on a student's ability to complete written tasks independently, not being able to put together sentences to describe something they have heard or know. Some connection is made, therefore, between structuring stories verbally and structuring them in a written form.

Unit 7   Assessment

Area of work: Listening to & retelling stories

Name of child:

Skills	Has this skill	Has demonstrated once in the group	Demonstrates regularly in the group	Has demonstrated outside the group
MAKING LINKS	✓	DATE	DATE	DATE
1 Can make one connection between two objects				
2 Can make one connection between two actions				
3 Can describe a sequence of three events				
TELLING STORIES				
4 Can identify what happens at the beginning, middle and end of a story				
5 Can name one identifying feature of a story character				
6 Can identify one significant prop for a story character				
7 Can identify significant aspects of a story setting				
8 Can translate the layout of a story scene on to the drama space				
9 Can retell a story using pre-sequenced props				
10 Can retell a story using pre-sequenced picture cards				
11 Can tell parts of a story in three steps				

Unit 7   Assessment *(Continued)*

Skills	Has this skill	Has demonstrated once in the group	Demonstrates regularly in the group	Has demonstrated outside the group
TELLING STORIES *(Continued)*	✓	DATE	DATE	DATE
12 Can tell a story in more than three steps				
13 Can tell a story using own combination of picture prompts				
14 Can create a story using combinations of prompts: pictures, words, props				
15 Can use simple narrative-drive words: *and, but, because*				
16 Can use a wider range of narrative-drive words				
LISTENING				
17 Can wait for turn to talk				
18 Can show interest in what others are saying by nodding head and using correct body position				
19 Can maintain a conversation by asking questions and using affirmatives				
20 Can extract key information in a story				

Notes

____

____

____

Unit 7　Aims

- ◉ To be able to make meaningful links between two or more things: objects, actions and events

- ◉ To develop thinking and commenting skills

- ◉ To learn a range of structural formats for telling stories.

Unit 7   Activities

Two-part stories

Perhaps the simplest story format is one where two things are linked together in a meaningful way. The next activities try to encourage this skill, using objects, actions and people. It is always helpful to repeat these activities, requiring a different combination each time, to demonstrate that different links between things are possible.

1 Things that go together

Starting at the simplest level, this activity aims to develop the capacity to recognise one connection between two things.

You need

A selection of everyday objects, ensuring that each has a possible pair, for example, bowl and spoon, toothbrush and toothpaste, hat and gloves. Make the links more or less obvious depending on the ability of the children.

Instruction

1 Spread out the objects and ask the children to find a pair.
2 Now ask them to make two sentences, saying what they are and what is their use: *'This is a ____ and a ____. They are used for ____'.*
3 Children share their sentences with the group.
4 Ask the children to find a new pair and make two more sentences.

2 Action/consequence

Donna Williams (1996) points out how important it is to be able to think about actions in terms of ordinary consequences for children with autism of any age.

You need

Suggestions for actions and their consequences (p211).

Instruction

1 Suggest an action to an individual group member or ask them to think of their own.
2 Provide an object needed to perform that action.
3 Tell the child to choose a partner and carry out the action.
4 The partner is provided with a consequence or can think of his own, but must respond to the action in a meaningful way.

Extension

Write out some actions and their possible consequences on separate cards. One child should hold up an action and a consequence card and the rest of the group should decide if this is a 'true or false' action/consequence.

3 Two people

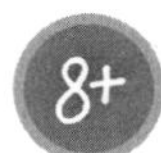

This activity encourages flexibility of thought around role.

You need

A selection of hats, masks and props that suggest different combinations of roles, for example, policeman's hat and robber's mask, nurse's hat and patient's bandage, school caps.

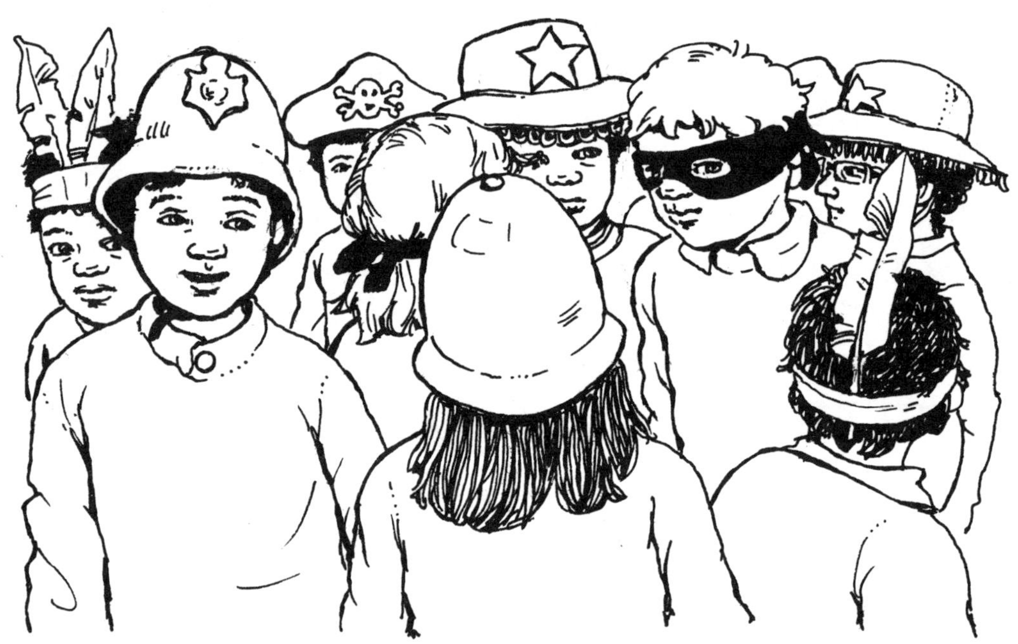

Instruction

1 Give group members one prop each.
2 Ask them to find someone who fits with their role.
3 When the children have paired up and established who they are, ask them to say or mime one typical activity they might do together.

4 One object, many actions

This activity encourages flexibility of thought around objects and actions.

You need

A selection of objects that have multiple uses, such as paper, a box, a chair or cloth.

Instruction

1 Pass the objects round the group asking each child to find a different way of using that object.
2 Tell them to make a sentence and mime an action as they use the object, *'I can ___ with a ___'*, substituting a different verb or verb phrase each time.

5 Body actions

A similar activity involves using parts of the body instead of objects.

Instruction

1 Focus on one body part in turn – hands, feet, eyes, head.
2 Find different verbs to describe what that part can do: *'I use my hands to wave'*, *'I use my head to nod "yes"'.*
3 Do not forget to include parts of the body that are not visible, especially the brain, to encourage the consideration of mental verbs (think, dream, work out).

These activities aim to encourage the use of a three-part storytelling format, to tell a simple story or to reduce a more complex story down to its component parts of beginning, middle and end. As with two-part stories, it is possible to link the work with a writing frame to support a piece of independent writing. The frame could take the form of two or three columns for subject + verb or subject + verb + object, or another three-part sentence.

6 Action sequences

Encourage children to create sequences of three in relation to stories and everyday actions.

You need

Blank cards, pens and a set of props.

Instruction

1   Brainstorm ordinary everyday activities such as making your bed, getting ready for school, going to the library.
2   Establish the activity in terms of three actions and draw onto cards or simply list, but number them 1–3.
3   Decide together on one prop to stand for each action sequence, such as a pillow for making the bed, schoolbag for getting ready for school, or library book.
4   Prompt each child to perform the action sequence by giving them the appropriate prop. For extra support, they can use the pictures or written list for that sequence.

7 Beginning/middle/end

Use a well-known story as the basis for the sequence of three.

You need

Three mats labelled *Beginning*, *Middle* and *End*.

Instruction

1   Choose a well-known story and read or tell it to the group.
2   Together establish what is the beginning, middle and end of the story.
3   Tell the children that they are going to create a sculpt or 'photograph' for each part.

4 Set out the labelled mats and get the children to move from mat to mat re-creating their sculpts.

5 Discuss together how successful the sculpt is in conveying the important details of that section of the story.

8 Topic/comment

This activity involves expanding on an agreed subject, thinking of different aspects or sequential steps.

Instruction

1 Decide on a topic such as making a journey, tidying your bedroom, making a cake, instructions for playing a game.

2 Do a round where children repeat the end of the previous statement and add an idea of their own, for example:
  - I went to the supermarket and bought some bread
  - I bought some bread, then I bought some bananas
  - I bought some bananas, then I looked at a magazine.

3 Create more sequences for other everyday activities.

These activities explore the basic components of a story: who, where and what. Before embarking on an activity, give some thought to the story you have chosen to use. In particular, consider what is its basic narrative structure. For example, does the narrative depend on a repetition of events as in *Goldilocks and the Three Bears*, or is it more about relational circumstances, such as in *Cinderella*, where the story is driven by the fact that Cinderella has no father, a wicked stepmother and two ugly sisters, and a good fairy godmother who helps her?

9 Who's knocking?

A fascinating activity which is surprisingly accessible to children with autism.

Instruction

1 After reading through a story, discuss the personalities and characters of the main characters.
2 Ask one child to leave the room and close the door.
3 The child should assume one character in the story and knock on the door in a style appropriate to that character.

10 Who am I?

This activity explores character through the use of a prop.

You need

One prop that is central to the story.

Instruction

1 Determine who are the main characters of a story.
2 Collect together props that are appropriate to those characters and to different parts of the story.
3 Set out a prop and ask the children to take it in turns to pick up and use it in the style of one of the characters.
4 The children can be given a character or choose one themselves which the group can then guess.

Variation

One child plays the main protagonist and the other children are secretly given a character to play. The protagonist must then greet and interact with each child until he can guess who they are.

11 Where diagrams

This activity develops the capacity to think about a story in relation to the space.

You need

A large blank sheet of paper and some pens.

Instruction

1 As a group, produce a floor plan for one scene in the story.
2 Use symbols to represent furniture, doors, windows, trees, water, whatever is relevant to the chosen scene.
3 Translate the plan to the space in the room by instructing individuals to go to different points indicated on the plan.
4 Pin up the plan so that the children can refer to it as they move around the space.

Extension

More able children can be instructed to go to an area and perform simple pretend actions: open the door, look out of the window, eat at the table. Props may be added to help with the improvisation.

12 What happened?

This activity moves into storytelling by combining the different aspects of a story outlined in the previous exercises.

You need

Three mats on the floor labelled *Who?*, *Where?* and *Doing what?*

Instruction

1 Tell the children they are going to retell a story by moving from mat to mat.
2 Give them a character (or they can select their own) and ask them to say who was where doing what, going from mat to mat.

Variation

Mats can have different labels depending on the format of the story you are using. For example, with *Goldilocks* you might use the labels *first*, *second* and *third*. For *Cinderella*, on the other hand, you might use the labels *Cinderella with whom?*, *Where?*, *Doing what?* More or less mats can be used depending on the ability and needs of the children.

The following activities give ideas about how to tell stories, using a variety of structures to prompt the recall and ease the retelling of stories. Some involve breaking down stories into their constituent parts, and you can use published materials to support this (see Useful Contacts at the end of the book). However, I find that an important part of the process of understanding stories is for pupils to make their own resources. As previously stated, a good prop box is handy.

13 Story cards

Make stories based on picture prompts.

You need

A set of blank cards or a published resource such as 'Combimage' (see Useful Contacts on p218).

Instruction

1 Brainstorm the typical elements of stories in terms of character, setting and objects.
2 Make a set of story cards, which could be colour coded according to these three categories, each card depicting one element.
3 Put all the cards in a row and ask individuals to pick out two, saying one connection between them.
4 Individuals could then pick out three (one of each colour) and make a sentence incorporating them.
5 Finally, ask individuals to make up their own stories choosing as many cards as they wish.

Variation

Do a similar activity, this time using props rather than story cards. Decide on a story and read it or tell it to the group. Using objects that relate to the different sections of the story, lay them out in the right order. Ask a child to retell the story using the objects.

14 Sound FX stories

Ask individual children to tell the story of their journey to school but using sounds instead of words.

Instruction

1 Establish the actual route of a child's journey to school and what happens or is seen along the way.
2 Agree what sound effects should be used for the journey.
3 Act out the journey using the agreed sound effects.
4 Add movement to show walking, stopping, turning the corner, going up or down, and so on.
5 Think of other routes and retell individually or in pairs.

Extension

Routes around a new school can be practised in this way.

15 Film storyboards

Use children's favourite films as the basis for storytelling.

You need

Storyboard template (p212).

Instruction

1 Decide on a film with which the children are familiar or one child's favourite film.
2 Briefly go through what happens in the film and then discuss in more detail what happens at the beginning, in the middle and at the end.
3 Explain that, as a group, you are going to create a storyboard for the film (you could show an example).
4 Choosing three or four significant scenes, sketch out a picture of what is happening to make a storyboard.
5 Use it to create a sculpt.
6 Consider the use of separate marked out areas and backdrops for each scene.
7 Some of the group as audience may then like to 'watch' the film being replayed.

In dramatherapy, there is a useful format for telling longer stories in six parts. It is based on the idea that many traditional stories conform to a structure of six basic elements which can be elicited by a set of questions (Lahad, 1992). Thinking of stories in six parts can move children with autism on from two- or three-part frames to more complex storytelling whilst continuing to provide a clear structure.

16 The six-part frame

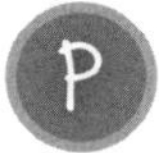

Use a writing frame to show children how even complex stories are constructed according to a format.

You need

Six-part story worksheet (p213).

Instruction

1   The children listen to a story – traditional ones work best – and then fill out the frame to give the six basic elements of the story.
2   Support for the work can be given by going through the story after it has been read, counting out the important elements.
3   The activity is repeated a few times so that different stories can be compared and the common themes and structures of stories highlighted.
4   Frames can then be used to help children to retell the stories.

It may seem odd to finish this unit with listening and yet, as a practitioner, I have found that listening – to really take in, understand and be able to respond – is the hardest task of all for children with autism. All the previous activities have concerned the skills of recalling and retelling events with a structure provided. These next activities aim to encourage the generation of new and original narratives or aspects of a narrative and probably require more in the way of skill.

17 Listening role play

Show 'good listening' and 'bad listening' in a role-played conversation, demonstrating each in turn.

Instruction

1 As a preliminary exercise, discuss what it means to listen.
2 Use role play to demonstrate good and bad listening and ask the children to say what it was that was right and wrong in the role play.
3 Ensure that some of the following points are made. In order to listen you need to:
   - sit still, face the speaker and not interrupt
   - try to remember what has been said and hold it in your mind
   - think about what the speaker is talking about
   - ask questions to get more information and continue the conversation
   - not change the subject or take over the conversation.
4 Once these points have been established, the children can take it in turns to practise conversations in the following activity.

18 One-minute listening

This is a fun way to think about listening which can be played in the style of a television game show.

You need

Each group member has a red card to hold.

Instruction

1 Two children, sitting in chairs and facing the group, role play a conversation; one is the speaker and one the listener.
2 The speaker decides on the topic and the conversation begins.

3 The group must judge how well the listener listens. In particular, they must look out for errors by the listener, for example, taking over the conversation, changing the subject from the agreed topic, or not asking enough questions for it to continue.
4 If a member of the audience spots an error, he or she can hold up their red card and explain what error the listener is making.
5 If they interrupt correctly, they can take on the role of listener. The listener wins if he or she manages to listen for one minute without interruption.

19 Gap stories

A challenging activity for both telling and listening to stories.

You need

Prompt boards for each group member with key storytelling words and phrases such as 'once upon a time', 'just then', 'bigger and bigger', 'happily ever after'.

Instruction

1 The group leader or a group member tells a story whilst the rest of the group listens.
2 The storyteller stops at significant places in the story to allow the listeners to add details: words or phrases taken from their prompt boards.
3 The storyteller must try to incorporate the listeners' ideas and still make a cogent story.

20 And, but, because

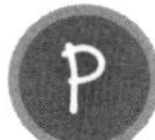 This activity practises children's use of narrative-drive words.

You need

A set of prompt cards showing narrative-drive words (p214).

Instruction

1 Put the cards face down in the middle of the group.
2 Begin to tell a story, stopping at a significant point.
3 The children take turns to pick a card and continue the story incorporating the word on the card.

Extension

Combine the story cards from Activity 13 with the word prompt cards from this activity. Ask the children to select a number of cards from each pile, for example, three story cards and one word card, and use them to make a story.

Improvisation 8

Putting experience and emotion together

Introduction

The ideas discussed in previous units, about carefully structuring learning, focusing on one thing at a time and gradually building a capacity for drama, come full circle when thinking about improvisation. Improvisation requires skills in pretence, interaction, storymaking and emotional expression but in a combined way that is much more sophisticated. One of the key issues in improvisation is the ability to create a 'representation' of experience, which is similar to what was discussed in Unit 3 in relation to sculpting, but this time expressing both external and internal states, the outward display and gestures of inner thoughts and feelings. Improvisation also requires the child to be 'in tune' with other performers, to respond to their actions and ideas and cooperate in some kind of storymaking. Particularly where the drama refers to typical events in a child's life, it also requires the ability to take a self-reflective stance and make self-narratives. Improvisation takes dramatic ability to a new level of spontaneity, creative thinking and communication.

In fact, there are high-functioning children with autism who relish the opportunity to do all of these things. I have known verbal, articulate children with Asperger Syndrome who have thrown themselves into improvised play. Workshop games, role play, acting out stories, improvising and putting on a performance can all be effective ways of working with such children. It is not the aim here to provide more ideas for this kind of dramatic work since there are plenty of good books on the subject. What will be explored, however, is how drama at this level can be particularly useful for developing aspects of social communication.

Drama offers unique opportunities for making sense of life to someone who struggles to understand the world around. Most importantly, it promotes the act of watching, both passively as part of the audience and more actively for those who are involved in the drama and must respond to what is happening. Drama makes it possible to watch situations of social interaction and communication as they occur, to analyse particular aspects and rehearse them. It provides a visible thinking aloud about social experience that can be slowed down, stopped, replayed, analysed and discussed. It could be said that life happens at too fast a pace for a child with autism, but using drama can allow someone to really see what is going on between two people.

Moreover, it is not all that clear that watching – being part of an audience – is merely a passive act. We are becoming increasingly aware that watching is in fact doing. In neuroscience, the discovery of mirror neurons has shown that parts of our brain are fired not only when we do something but also when we *watch* someone do something (Gallese, 2001). Augusto Boal, the great theatre director and political activist, touches on a similar phenomenon when he argues that the very act of watching drama can 'dynamise' an individual so that he feels more able to express and act himself in situations related to a scene (Boal, 1992).

○ Playback Theatre

Boal's ideas relate to a form of community theatre, usually known as improvisational theatre, which has less to do with any scripted tradition of drama and more with the issues of daily life of the participants. Boal founded Forum Theatre as a way of bringing drama to the streets to address issues of culture and oppression, but there are other forms of improvisational theatre that also exist. Playback Theatre, for example, developed by Jonathon Fox in the 1970s, provides a particularly clear format that is easy to use with groups of children.

In Playback, one person volunteers to be a 'teller' and tells a story to the group, the 'actors', about something that has happened to him. The group then acts out the story whilst the teller watches. The space is set out simply, delineating areas for the teller to watch, for the actors to sit and for the acting area itself. Simple props may be to hand on a 'prop tree'. Stories should concern something that has happened recently or in the past and may relate a particular incident or something that happens every day. The acting area is mapped in relation to the story so that everyone is clear what happens where. Discussion follows the enactment and the teller is asked to give feedback on the accuracy of the representation. The incident itself might also be discussed:

- How did the participants in the event feel?
- Why did they say and do the things they did?
- What might they have been done differently?
- What did someone say that was effective?

For a child with autism, Playback provides a straightforward way of going back over something that has happened and thinking about what really went on. Looking again at an incident, and in such a visual way, allows the child to grasp more fully what happened and the feelings that were involved, including his own emotional reactions. The incident may be something that happens regularly but is hard to understand, something he did well, or something that is a problem. The subject matter could be similar to that used for a social story or comic strip conversation as devised by Carol Gray (1997). Discussion helps to point out what is the right or expected response in a situation – what you would normally do – as well as what is not a social norm. Moreover, freeze framing a scene allows the child to see the physical expressions that were adopted at the time and to have their non-verbal meaning explained.

The following activities focus on the child's capacity to improvise, initially through simple one-off acts of improvisation and later through more sophisticated and reciprocal group exchange. They serve to develop the skills needed to use Playback, which is explained in more detail. Finally, other ways of exploring social issues are provided.

Unit 8   Assessment

Area of work Improvisation

Name of child

Skills	Has this skill	Has demonstrated once in the group	Demonstrates regularly in the group	Has demonstrated outside the group
SINGLE ACTS	✓	DATE	DATE	DATE
1 Makes effective use of hands, body, face and the dramatic space when miming objects				
2 Can use abstract objects in creating a pretence				
3 Can relate pretend objects to each other				
4 Can combine a pretend action with a given adverb				
5 Can represent an inner feeling state through combined use of body, face and posture				
6 Can combine a pretend action with an inner feeling state				
7 Can make exits and entrances				
RECIPROCAL ACTS				
8 Can synchronise self with partner when being mirrored				
9 Can mirror with fluency another person's movement, gesture, walk and vocal expression				
10 Can share pretend objects				

Skills	Has this skill	Has demonstrated once in the group	Demonstrates regularly in the group	Has demonstrated outside the group
RECIPROCAL ACTS *(Continued)*	✓	DATE	DATE	DATE
11 Can join in with pretend actions				
12 Can adopt recognisable mannerisms and traits of a fictional character				
13 Can speak a given line with expression in a dialogue				
14 Can re-enact a given scene in role within a group				
15 Can adopt a variety of roles				
CAPACITY FOR REFLECTION				
16 Can state the probable intentions and reactions of a character in a scene				
17 Can provide a line of dialogue for a character in a scene				
18 Can react in words and actions to another child's improvisation				
19 Can adapt improvised material following discussion				
20 Can comment on a re-enactment saying what feelings and ideas it evokes				

Notes

____

____

____

◉ To be able to carry out pretend acts conveying both outward appearance and internal feeling states

◉ To be able to imagine what a character might say or feel

◉ To be able to respond in role within an improvisation

◉ To be able to reflect on an improvisation and draw realistic parallels with real life and own experience.

Unit 8   Activities

The emphasis here is on expressing an inner state of mind through outward gestures in single non-reciprocal acts of improvisation. The aim is to develop the child's improvisational expression, creativity and spontaneity.

1 Object rhythms

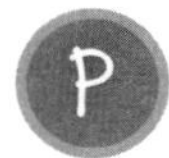

This is a classic Viola Spolin (1986) activity that is good for warming up the body and imagination.

You need

See Mime ideas (p203).

Instruction

1 Ask the children to walk around the room, using all the space and trying not to make eye contact with each other.
2 Tell them that when you call out an object, they should stop and mime using it.
3 Instruct them that they should continue experimenting with their mime until they are happy with it, when it has a rhythm and flow to it and can be easily be repeated.
4 When the children are happy with their mime, they can walk around the room again performing their object rhythm.
5 After a while and whilst they are still walking, tell the children to wipe out their mime using their hands and wait for the next object to be named.

Extension

You can combine an object with an adjective to evoke more feeling in the mime, for example, eating hot food, putting on tight trousers. Alternatively, combine an object with a situation such as making a 999 call, cutting out paper to wrap a present, getting dressed to go to a party.

2 Space shaping

An alternative warm-up activity for body and imagination.

Instruction

1 Children should stand in an area by themselves and focus their attention on the space in front of them.
2 Tell them to allow their hands, arms and body to move freely within the space and see if an object or action takes form.

3 When it does, children should be encouraged to explore it, to see how big,
   how tall, how heavy it is, what it feels like in terms of touch, whether it
   moves if you touch it, how much force you need to push it.

Comment

This activity is also from the work of Viola Spolin (1986) who points out that
children must be encouraged to move their whole body and not stand rigidly
moving their arms. Only in this way will an object take substance and seem
authentic rather than forced upon the space. She advises giving constant
reminders to children about what they should be doing and thinking including:

- 'Keep track of the object'
- 'Give the object enough room in space'
- 'Keep the object in space – not in your head!' (Spolin, 1986).

3 Object changing emotion

By combining action with emotion, children need to consider both
inner feeling and outer appearance.

You need

See suggestions for object changing emotion situations (p215).

Instruction

1 Give each child an idea for an improvisation, telling them an object and a
   situation where their feeling about the object changes.
2 Individuals take turns to do a mime, performing to the group so that other
   children have the opportunity to view the improvisation, and the
   facilitator can provide more in the way of support.

4 Just before

A simple yet effective improvisation which can reveal much about
how emotions are conveyed by the body.

Instruction

1 Give the children a suggestion of something they might have just done, such
   as running because they were late, arguing with a friend, being given an *A+*
   mark.
2 Suggestions can be whispered or written down.

3   Individuals then go out of the room and re-enter it, joining the group in
    such a way that communicates what they were doing just before they came
    in.
4   The group must guess what it is.

Variation

Instead of showing what you have just finished doing, the children can be asked
to express their anticipation of something that will happen 'next'.

Comment

Some children with autism have difficulty understanding time and with how to
relate experience in a temporal way. These activities are a good way of teaching
the concepts of *before, earlier, now, next* and *then*.

Improvisation in pairs

Some children with autism show no preference when working with another child in a pair, for them one child being much the same as another. Doing improvised paired work in a group, where two children together are encouraged to be creative and receptive to each other's ideas, can be an effective way of working. I have known friendships to emerge from such an experience, but careful consideration is necessary about who to pair with whom.

5 Walk my walk

An activity which plays with the idea of putting yourself in another person's shoes.

Instruction

1 Put the children into pairs and have the whole group sit along one side of the room.

2 Tell the children to watch one member of the group walk around the space in a circle.

3 Encourage them to consider what the child is doing in terms of his body: are his shoulders up or down, how does he use his feet, what is the pace and rhythm of his walk?

4 Ask his partner to copy his walk by first standing a little bit behind and to one side. The pair should walk around the room, in a large circle as before, with the second child learning his partner's walk.

5 When the partner feels he has learned it, he nods his head and the first child sits down. That child then watches whilst his partner walks his walk.

Variation

You can substitute walking with talking. Partners sit side by side having agreed what one will say, either the exact words or the gist of the talk. One child then begins talking whilst his partner tries to say what he is saying at exactly the same time.

Comment

Once they are aware of their partner's walk or talk, encourage the children not to look at their partner but to have a feel for what he is doing. More than simply mimicking, sensing people provides a more powerful way of 'getting inside them' and is aided by not directly looking.

6 Who is the mirror?

This activity is a more skilful form of partner mirroring described in Unit 3.

Instruction

1 Pairs should face each other, one child instructed to copy the other's movements as if he were looking in a mirror.
2 The lead child should be considerate to their partner and try not to move too quickly.
3 You can use music to help the children's movements flow.
4 Allow the children to swap roles, so that they have turns to be leader.
5 Eventually, when a partnership is working well, the partner who follows can almost anticipate what the leader will do, as if they are moving as one person. It is possible to eventually lose the sense that one person is leading and the other following, when the instruction 'No leader' is possible.

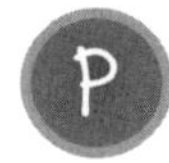

7 Parts of a whole

This activity practises the skill of joining in with another person's imaginative idea.

You need

Suggestions for mime ideas (p203).

Instruction

1 Put the children into pairs or ask them to choose a partner.
2 Instruct one child to choose an activity and mime it, asking them to repeat it until a rhythm is established.
3 Give the partner plenty of time to watch the mime and consider how he will participate in it.
4 He must then join in with the activity in some way that is appropriate to the original mime.

Variation

This activity can be done with or without the partner knowing what is being mimed. It can also be done with or without dialogue.

8 Asking for the ball

Asking for your ball to be returned provides a short scene with lots of potential.

You need

A foam ball.

Instruction

1 Children in pairs are asked to improvise a short scene where one child must ask for his football which he has accidentally kicked over his neighbour's fence.
2 The child who is playing the neighbour is given a character or role, for example, a person who is hard of hearing, a very tall person, a child, a policeman or a witch.
3 Give the pair a short time to prepare their improvisation and then ask them to show it.
4 The first child must knock on his neighbour's door and ask for the ball and the neighbour should respond in role.
5 The audience should guess what it is.

9 I say, you say

An effective way of combining feeling with the spoken word.

You need

Reciprocal lines that have an emotive or conflictual quality such as:

- I can't – Yes, you can
- I don't understand you – You do understand me
- Be my friend – I'm not your friend
- Give it to me – You can't have it.

Instruction

1 Put the children into pairs and give each child one line to say.
2 Partners stand at either end of the room and say the lines to each other over and over, trying to give them as much expression as possible.
3 Encourage expression by specifying how the lines should be said, for example, gently, pleadingly, desperately, coldly, lovingly.

Here are more straightforward ideas for improvisation, but this time carried out by the whole group.

10 Tug-of-war

A physical warm-up for the whole group.

You need

A line marked out on the floor.

Instruction

1 Divide the group and ask one child to pick a partner of equal strength from the other group.
2 Instruct the pair to try to pull each other over the line, but without actually touching or using a rope.
3 The pair can decide beforehand how they are going to play the game, deciding, for example, who will be the winner.
4 When the children are familiar with the improvisation, add more players to each side, building up a whole group tug-of-war.

11 My favourite game

This activity has a similar format to the Playback work that follows.

Instruction

1 Set out two chairs, one for the facilitator and one for a child.
2 Have the rest of the group sit facing with a space between.
3 The child is asked to name his favourite game, explaining how he understands it is played.
4 The facilitator goes over what the child has said, emphasising the rules and pointing to areas within the acting space that relate to it.
5 The group is asked to re-enact the game, being given or deciding themselves on their role within it.
6 The child watches the group re-enact his favourite game and gives feedback at the end on how authentic the improvisation felt.
7 Another child then has a turn to have his favourite game re-enacted.

12 We say

This is a line repetition exercise with the involvement of the whole group.

You need

Sets of reciprocal lines, as used for Activity 9, 'I say, you say'.

Instruction

1 Divide the group and ask them to line up along two walls facing each other.
2 Give each side a line to say and a way in which to say it, for example, quietly, angrily, nervously.
3 Tell them to repeat their lines to each other, expressing them as emotively as possible.

13 Party

Lots of fun can be had with this short scene about arriving at a party.

You need

Blank cards, a pen and a doorbell.

Instruction

1 As a group, brainstorm different characters who might go to a party. Ideas can be straightforward, such as a friend, your teacher, a stranger, or they can be more imaginative such as Father Christmas, an alien, someone who is gradually turning into a monster.
2 Characters can be written out on cards and the children given one by picking a card.
3 They should think about what that character might be like: his or her typical mannerisms, expression, things to say, and so on.
4 One child is the party host and answers the doorbell to each guest.
5 The guest should greet the host and join the party in a way suggested by his character.
6 The host or audience can guess who the guest is.

Variation

Each child is given or thinks of an occupation. They line up as if waiting for a bus, standing, fiddling and interacting with each other, in a way that suggests their occupation. The improvisation can be carried out by any number of children with other group members watching and guessing the occupation.

Playback

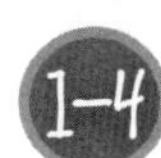

Structuring improvisation along the lines of Playback Theatre provides a straightforward and effective way of re-enacting scenes from a child's life. Scenes may be re-enacted for the purpose of exploring something with which the child is having difficulty, or where he has succeeded. The facilitator may decide the content of the improvisation and invite the child to relate what happened when. In this instance, improvisation is used as a resource for understanding more about social situations, for learning life skills and developing new ways of interacting and communicating. Playback structure can be used in a less directed way, however, where group members are asked simply to share something about themselves with the rest of the group, the exercise contributing more to the development of trust, self-esteem and group reciprocity.

In Playback, the space is used in a set way, with a designated acting area, chairs for the facilitator and child whose story is being re-enacted, chairs or boxes for the actors, a place for the audience and a container for simple props (see Figure 8.1). If the group is small so that all members must be actors and involved in the improvisation, it is possible to dispense with an audience. In fact, the child storyteller and the facilitator are an audience in themselves.

You need

Chairs or boxes for each participant and a prop box set out as shown in Figure 8.1.

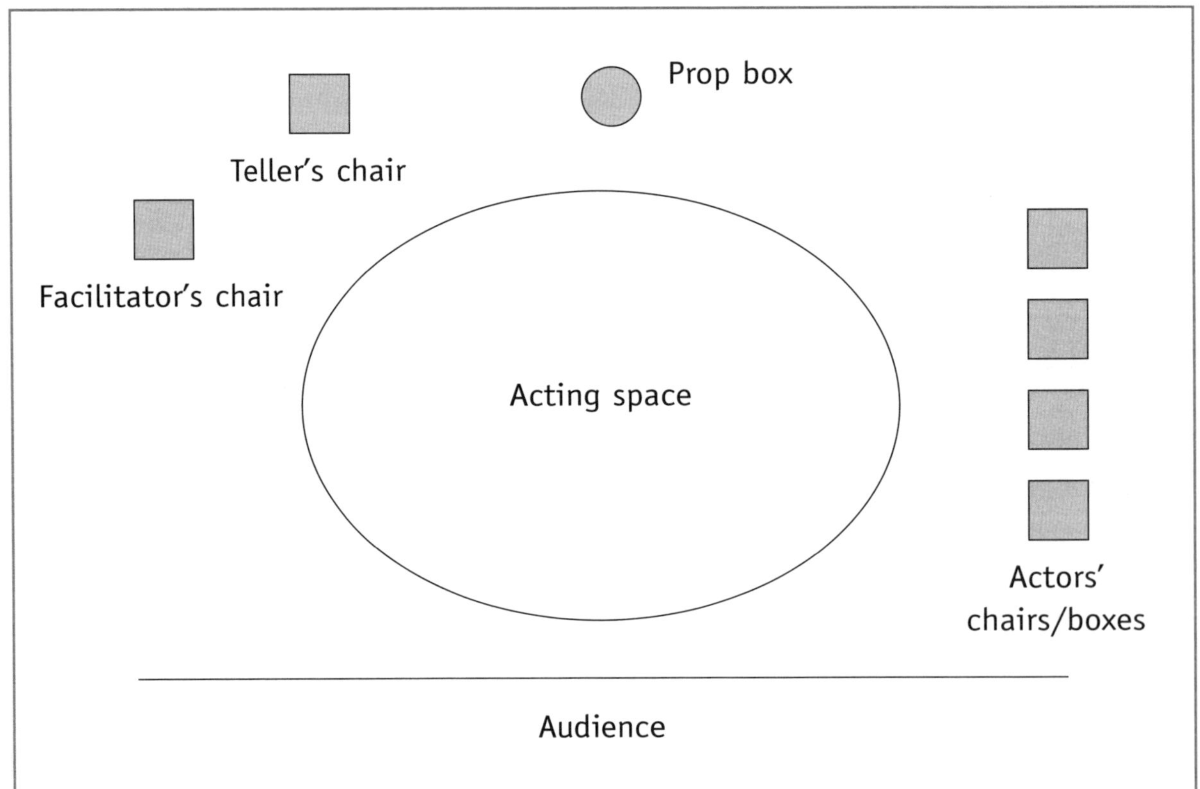

Figure 8.1 Organisation of Playback Theatre space

 USING DRAMA WITH CHILDREN ON THE AUTISM SPECTRUM

14 The story: step one

Invite one child to sit beside you in the teller's chair. You may ask the children for a volunteer or you may name a child. If you want to use Playback to go over something specific that has happened, you can ask the child to describe what happened. Sometimes it is helpful to have a chat first, as a way of breaking the ice, before getting on to the business in hand. If there is no specific event for the improvisation, you can simply ask a child to tell a story about something that has happened.

Once the story has been told, you should go over the sequence of events with the teller, numbering them on your fingers. Ask for clarification on any parts of it that are not clear and ask questions to elicit parts of the story not fully told. If other children in the group know about the incident they can contribute at this point, but you should emphasise that this is the teller's version of events. Go over the story sequence again, this time for the benefit of the whole group so that everyone is clear about where the story begins and ends and what they need to do.

15 The actors: step two

Establish who is involved in the story and how many characters there are, and set out an appropriate number of chairs in the actors' space. Ask for volunteer actors or select particular children yourself. Specify which actor's seat belongs to which character and invite the child actor to sit in it. When all the actors are seated, ask them if

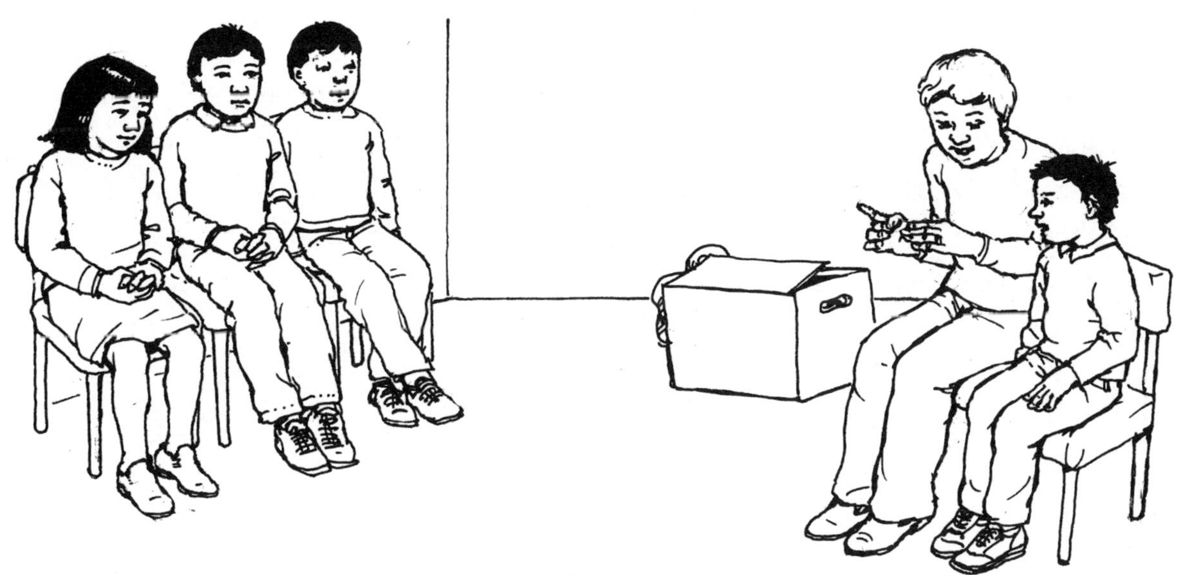

there is anything they wish to clarify with the teller about the story. You may also go over the story one more time so that the actors know what their character needs to do.

16 The improvisation: step three

The actors prepare for the improvisation by setting out any furniture or props they need, using their chairs and the prop box. They then act out the story using the acting space. Inform the teller that he should just watch at this stage and will have the opportunity to comment at the end of the re-enactment.

17 The discussion: step four

When the re-enactment is finished, ask the teller to give feedback. How accurate was it? Is there anything he would like to see done differently? How did watching it make him feel? The teller can also be asked why the story is important to him. At this point, the incident itself can also be discussed. If the Playback activity is aimed at addressing a particular behaviour in the child or an area of understanding, you can explore issues related to what was actually happening. You can ask the actors to go back over a particular moment and ask questions about how a character felt and why he did or said something. In order to explore emotional communication more deeply, you can freeze the action and point out a character's non-verbal body language and facial expression, or you can touch characters on the shoulder, asking them what they are thinking and feeling.

Following the discussion, some conclusions may be drawn about what was depicted. You can point out where things went wrong for the child and what he might do next time, or you may tell him what he did that was right. You may ask the teller to think about how he feels now about what happened. Ask him to focus on himself, to locate the feeling and to try to give it a word or phrase.

Billy, aged 13, told a story about an incident at home where he had argued with his sister and his mum, and had got really angry. He told the group that he had been playing with his sister and her two friends in her bedroom, but that he had got upset because they would not play the game properly. He said they were chatting and being silly and he had felt excluded. In his frustration, he had picked up an ornament and thrown it, smashing it in the process. When his mother came to see what was going on, she got angry with him but not with his sister or the friends, which Billy thought was unfair. The group acted out the scene and, in the way the characters sat and interacted, Billy's excluded position could be clearly seen. In the discussion that followed, it emerged that the mother's response to Billy's actions might have been based on what she knew about him from previous incidents. Billy was asked to focus on how he felt when he got upset and threw the ornament and asked to put it into words. Billy said that he realised something now and had a word to explain what was happening for him, the word being `Control'. Together, the group brainstormed things that Billy could have done instead of getting upset.

It is not always necessary to go too deeply into the improvisation, particularly where the child has volunteered a story and just wants to share it with the group. However, try to explore issues of friendship and social understanding that relate to children other than the child with autism so that that child is not always the focus of the work, and as a way of demonstrating that we all struggle with these difficult issues.

Improvisation to explore social issues

There are many ways of using improvisation to explore social issues. Here are just a few.

18 Letter to an alien

This activity plays with the idea of explaining social issues to someone from another planet who has no understanding of the ways of human beings.

You need

Paper, blank cards, pen, coloured pencils, scissors, interesting photographs and pictures, magazines.

Instruction

1 Create a collage or words and pictures on a chosen theme, such as friendship, school, family, play.
2 The idea is that the collage should explain the theme to someone who is not from planet Earth and does not have a human understanding of such things.

19 Social sculpts

This activity explores social situations and feelings imaginatively and creatively.

Instruction

1 In groups of three or four, ask the children to create a sculpt to depict a social issue and what that means to them. Topics could be such things as friendship, bullying, satisfaction, anger.
2 The image created could be based on an actual incident or could try to convey some more abstract and collective idea.
3 Tell the groups they have ten minutes to create the sculpt and, when they are ready, can take turns to show them to the group.
4 The audience can each give one word to describe what they think is being depicted.

Extension

Audience members are invited to stand beside one 'character' in the sculpt and supply a word of dialogue or say what that person might be thinking.

20 My life as a film

Many children love films and the idea of creating one of their own based on their lives is very appealing.

Instruction

1 Organise the children into groups of two or three, one person volunteering to use their life as the basis for a sculpt.
2 He should choose a small number of significant events from his life and think of a title for his 'film'.
3 His group then create a scene or tableau for each event, presenting snapshots of his life.
4 They present it to the whole group.

Introduction

It is vital to have a definite point of ending in drama, where participants are able to disengage from whatever pretence has been created and move from a dramatic world back to the real one. A clear ending is important because it is not always easy to make that transition, especially where what has been imaginatively created *feels* real. Actors talk of not being able to shake off a character or mood that came upon them whilst engaged in a drama. Similarly, with children, the realism within drama can create a 'high' and teachers know they must incorporate 'winding down' activities to close a drama lesson.

In drama, there are a number of customary ways of ending a session. Jones (1996) points out that in a theatre performance the applause of the audience and return to the stage of the actors is one such way, marking the end of the story and taking off of all roles. Other ways of ending include closing the curtains of the performance space, packing away props and removing costumes. Dramatherapy uses 'de-roling' exercises such as physically brushing off or washing off a role, reconnecting with the here and now by noticing actual details of the room and the people in it, or taking time for individuals to connect with their real selves by relating some personal details. The process of discussing the impact of the drama on the individual participants will also serve the purpose of bringing them back to themselves. For younger children, it is possible to bring the session to a close by tidying up and putting things away, or by addressing simple questions to individual children about what they have just done and by taking the time to say goodbye.

○ The significance of transitions in autism

The idea of a transition, from 'pretend experience' to 'real experience', does raise a question where autism is concerned. Children with autism often experience the real world and the people in it as alien and unreal. Alternatively, others live permanently in a fantasy world, which they find impossible to give up. The nature of autism often means a poor grasp of and inflexibility about any notion of 'pretend'. How then does one provide an effective ending to drama?

Autism involves a lack of any overall understanding of social experience, in particular, an inability to distinguish one experience from another, to know when it has ended and the next begun. Children with autism often seem at sea in a social world, experiences washing over them without making a singular impact in terms of meaning. Anyone working with autism will know the importance of routines and the anxiety caused by disruptions to the norm. This is why a visual timetable works so well in reducing anxiety and calming down behaviour. 'Finished' is a key factor here, with the act of putting away the symbol card that denotes an activity giving a concrete experience that it has come to an end and something else is about to begin.

○ How to work with endings

Working with endings must be part of the overall programme as well as of every session of drama for children with autism. An effective ending to a session will serve the purpose of clearly delineating pretend from real life as well as helping with the understanding of ending per se. However, whilst it is possible to incorporate some ending activities typically used in drama, it may be necessary to make adaptations or give a different emphasis. Some children with autism are not able to invest that much in the way of imaginative projection in the first place, and endings need to focus less on bringing them out of their imaginative world and back to real life and more on giving a clear visual experience of 'the end'. For other children, who have a rich imagination or who have participated fully in pretence, other more familiar forms of ending drama will be appropriate.

The following activities suggest ways of ending individual sessions as well as how to bring to a close a group that has run for a length of time. In both cases, the aim of the work is twofold: to provide a clear indication that the group work has come to end whilst enabling children to reflect a little on what they have achieved. In this way, children should both be clear about the fact of ending as well as able to gain some satisfaction from and understanding of what they have just done.

Unit 9   Activities

1 Providing information

A simple way of working with endings is to provide information about the details of the session: how long it will be, what time it will finish, where the children will go next and what they will do then. You can also outline what will happen in the session itself, what they will be working on and the sequence of activities. At the end, you can specify when you will see them again and, if it is a regular slot, whether there is any change to the usual arrangements. If there is a change, count down the days or weeks to it, giving the children plenty of warning. Once you have outlined the details, make sure you stick to them and do not go against the plans you have described.

2 Ending rituals

Good practice when working with children dictates both beginning and ending rituals, which may be similar in content. A ritual can be almost anything which is done regularly to mark a particular moment. Rituals for young children may be singing a special song or saying goodbye to each child in turn. Older and more able children may like to play a familiar game or circle time activity.

3 Feedback

A plenary at the end of sessions can become an ending ritual. Children are asked to go over what they just did and, with more able children, to reflect on their achievements. Children can be invited to say something about the session or say one thing they will take from it. They may be asked to say what they did well, what they liked about what another child did or what their favourite activity was. It is important for the facilitator to point out something that has been learned through the drama, particularly some aspect of social learning. Parallels with everyday life may be drawn to help generalise the learning that has taken place in the group.

4 Clearing away the space

Perhaps the most effective ending for children with autism is the actual clearing of the drama space, the putting away of any toys and props that have been used. Clearing away gives a concrete message that the activity is finished and, once the space is cleared, gives a strong visual message too. You can ask the group of children to help set out the space, the chairs, props, set – whatever is required for the session – and then ask them to clear it away at the end, again a clear indication of a beginning and an ending.

5 De-roling

For some children, de-roling will be an important form of ending. De-roling involves 'taking off' the role or character that the child has played and should involve the whole body. A role is something that is physically taken on and should be taken off in a way that is physical too. Children can wash off or brush off a role, brushing down their limbs. You can demonstrate how to take on a role and de-role by stepping in and out of an acting space saying 'Here I am as me. Here I am as a policeman. Here I am as me again', adopting suitable body posture and demeanour each time. Sometimes it is important to point out a child's *humanity* in the act of de-roling: 'My name is Tom and I'm a boy.' For a child who needs this level of de-roling, however, the whole enterprise of adopting roles should be carefully considered, with ample use of structure.

<u>**Activities for when the group ends**</u>

You should think carefully about how to end a group that has been meeting regularly and working together for some weeks. The purpose of the final or final few sessions is to make a note of the end and to celebrate the achievements of the members of the group, but also to help the children take leave of each other in the group.

6 Talking about the end

The ending of a group should be present in the beginning, with clarity about the purpose, make-up and form of the group, as well as its duration. Occasionally, specify how many sessions remain as a way of counting down to the end and preparing the children for it. Look forward to the future, when the group has ended, by talking about what the children will be doing at that time of the week.

7 Celebration

Discuss with the children what they would like to do in the last session. You can plan it with them, the children naming favourite activities they would like to repeat in the last session, or you can use the last session for a party. Again, plan it together, thinking about what you want to do: will there be food, will the children get dressed up, how will you decorate the room? Some children like to be asked to do a party 'turn', perhaps repeating a talent they have already demonstrated in the group. In any case, the end session should be a celebration of the group itself, and of the individuals in it. Children can be asked to say:

- one thing they remember from the group
- one important thing they have learned
- one thing they have learned from another child in the group.

The facilitator can take the opportunity to point out good things to the children about themselves, to give awards for achievement and generally praise and celebrate the group's achievements.

8 Personal albums

Where a child has achieved, particularly in terms of social skill, self-esteem and self-awareness, you might like to make an album for him showing those achievements. The album can take the form of photographs or cartoons stating what the child has done and learned, or describing positive sides of his character that he has demonstrated in the group. Write about the child in clear, affirmative sentences that begin 'You can...' and 'You are...'. During the group, you may make a note of particular achievements and record these in a personal album, writing 'I remember that you...'.

9 The line

In the final session, you can ask the children to consider the future and how they will act and think differently as a result of being in the group. You can give them a concrete image of the future by marking out a white line on the floor. Ask children what they think is on the other side of the line. What will they do or say differently having been in and learned from the group? How do the children feel about the future? What are they looking forward to? Invite the children to approach and step over the line in a manner that reflects their feelings about the future.

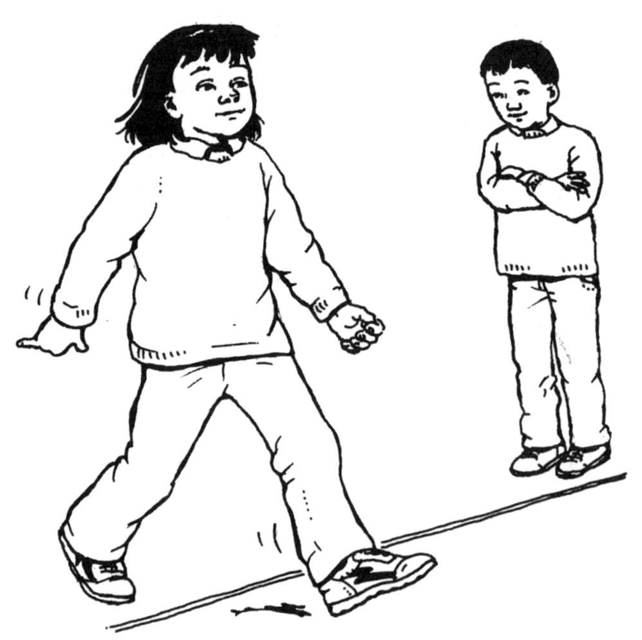

APPENDICES

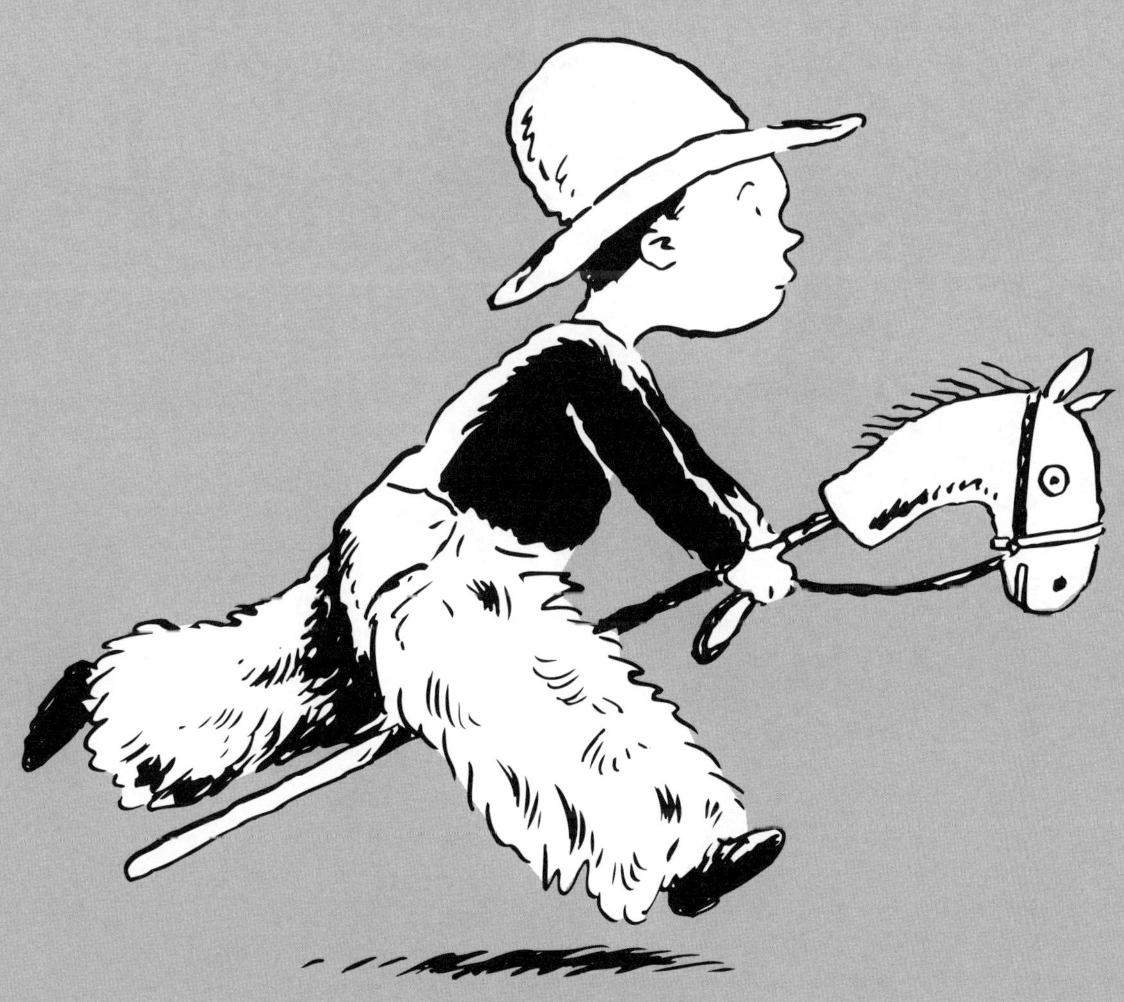

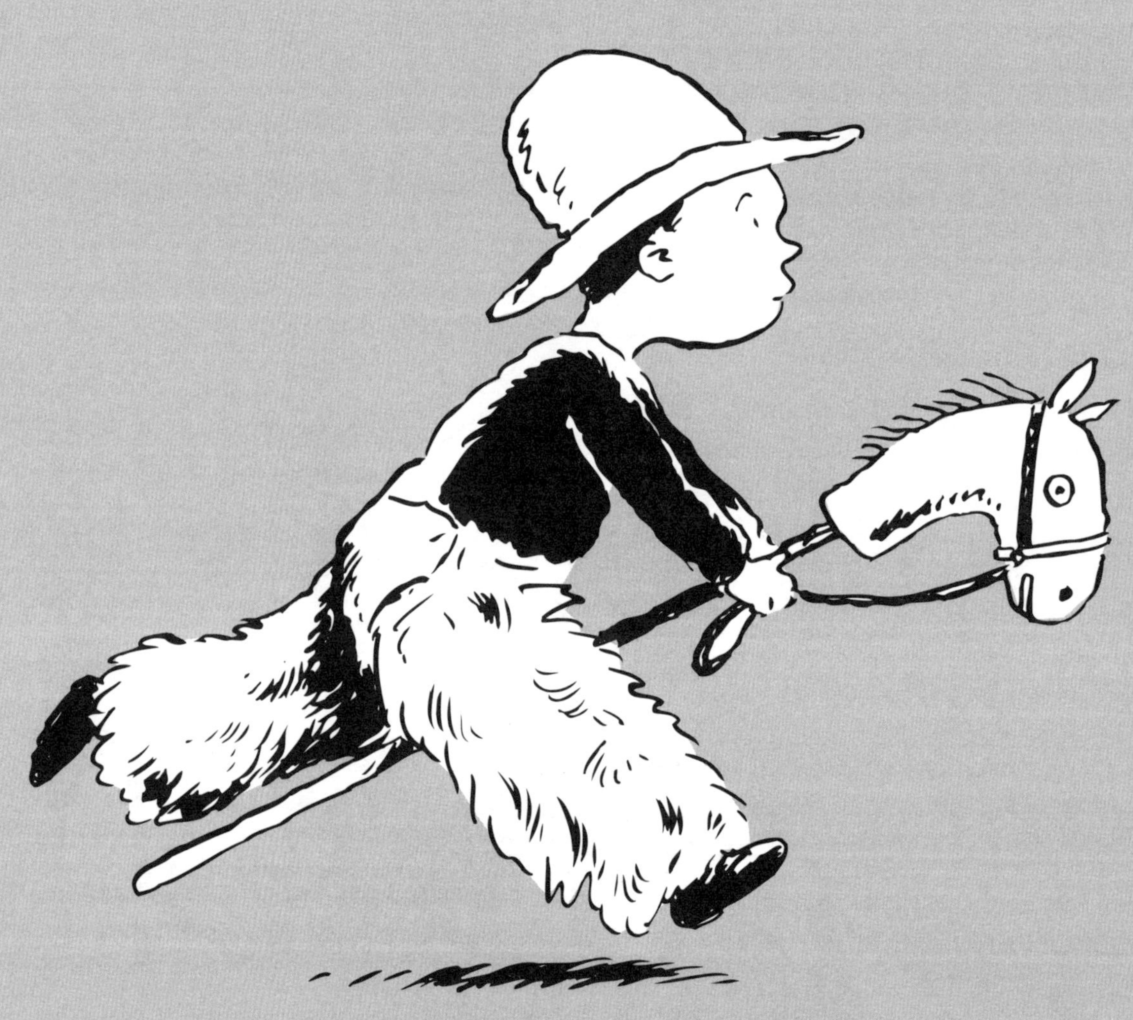

List of Appendices

Appendix I

Mime ideas

(Unit 3 Activity 13; Unit 8 Activities 1 & 7)

Tossing a pancake
Painting at an easel
Stroking a cat
Looking for something (specify what)
Getting dressed
Watering the garden
Tidying up your bedroom
Taking a shower
Putting rubbish in the bin
Making a sandwich
Playing a computer game (specify)
Shaking hands and saying hello
Looking after a toddler
Putting on a DVD
Arranging flowers
Rollerblading
Keeping a balloon in the air
Eating an ice-cream
Washing up
Making a phone call
Cutting with scissors
Playing with playdough
Eating spaghetti
Playing with a ball (specify game)

Movement and sound words

(Unit 3 Activity 16; Unit 5 Activity 8)

1 Movement words	2 Sound words
Hop	Buzz
Shake	Click
Stamp	Cough
Nod	Beep
Stretch	Whoop
March	Hiss
Blink	Whizz
Crawl	Swish
Wiggle	Gasp
Shuffle	Hum

Scene cards

(Unit 3 Activities 17 & 18; Unit 4 Activity 20)

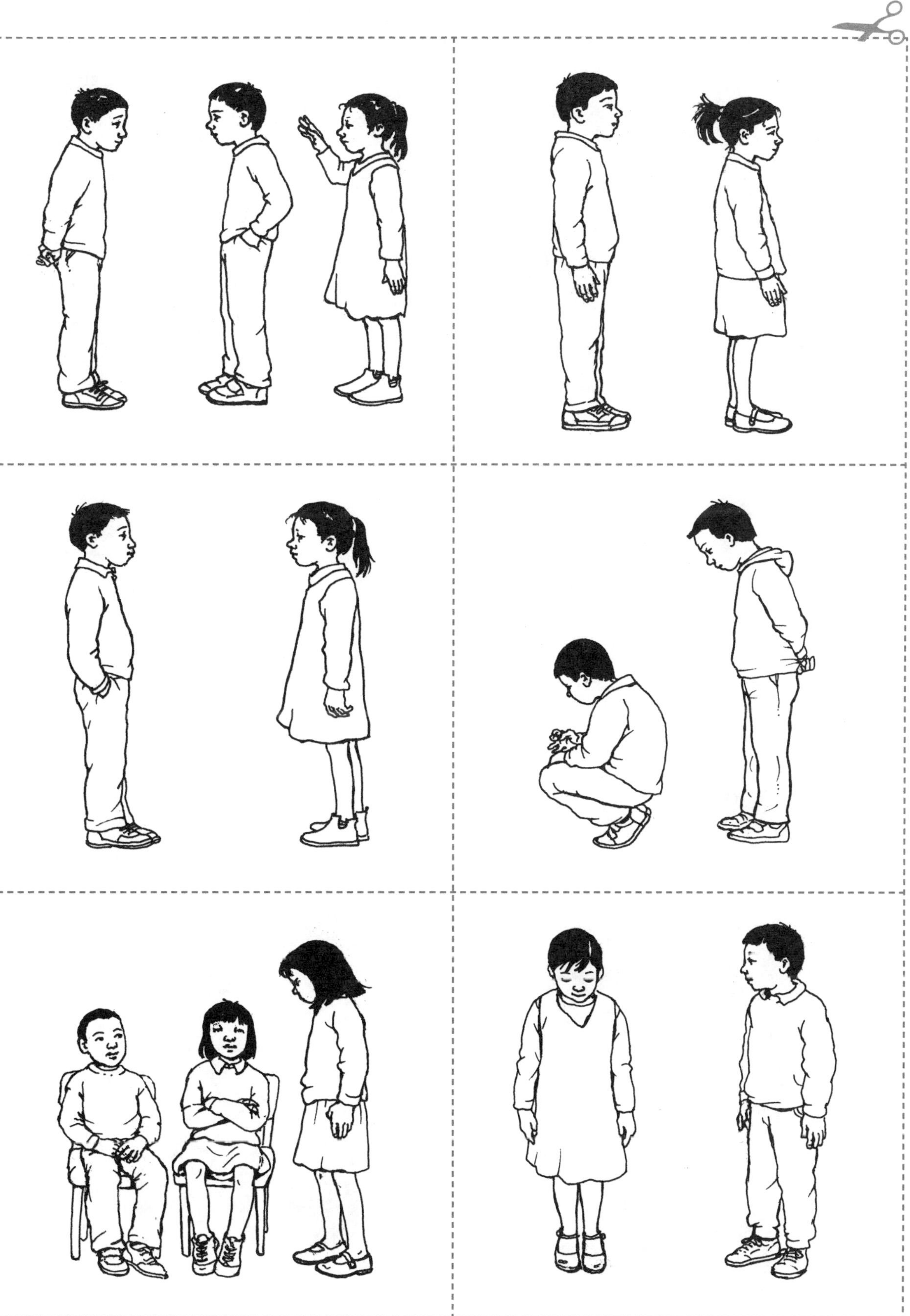

Scene cards

(Unit 3 Activities 17 & 18; Unit 4 Activity 20)

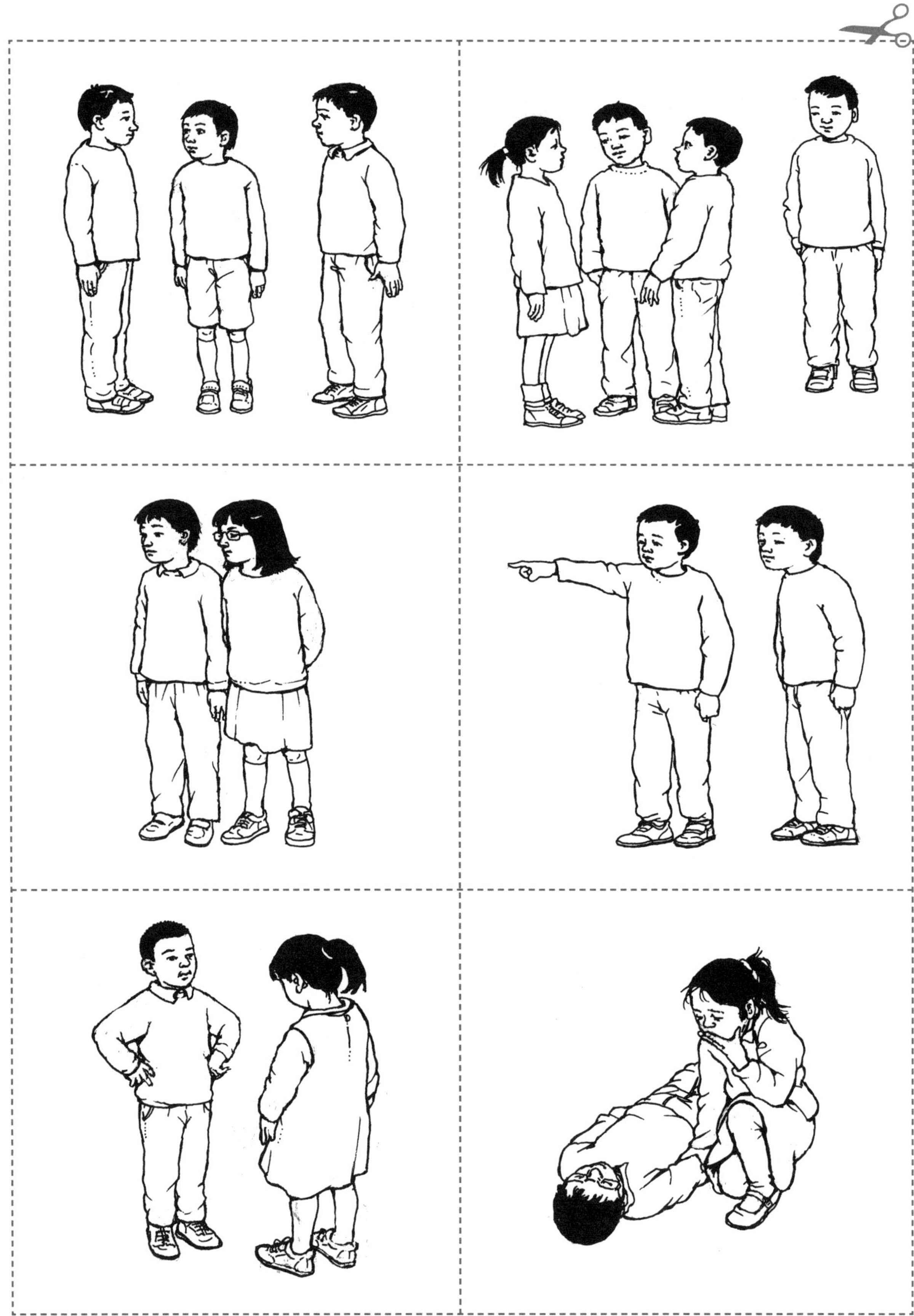

Volume gauge

(Unit 4 Activities 7 & 9)

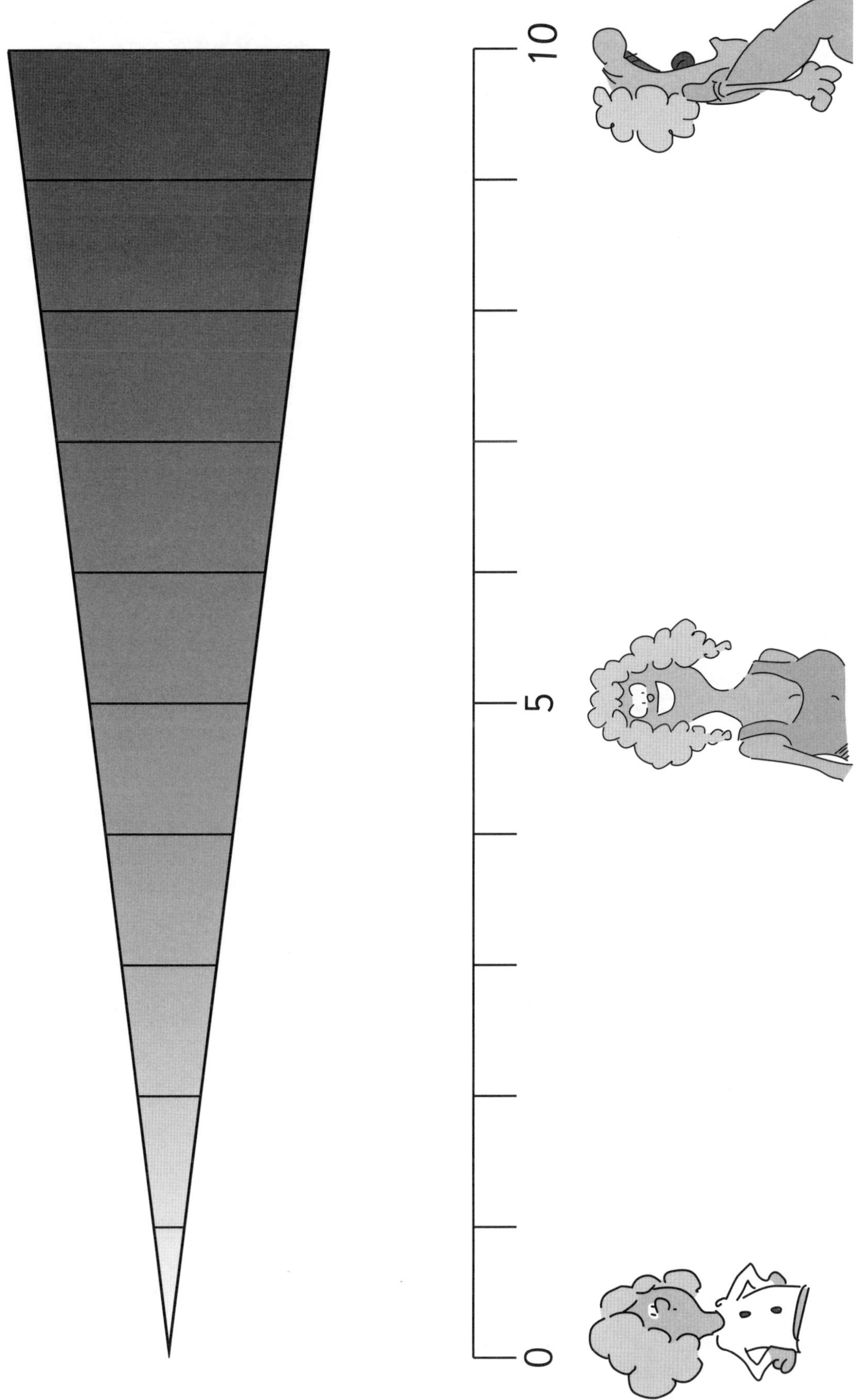

Sets

(Unit 5 Activity 5)

Knife	It is made of metal	It is used for cutting
Cup	It has a handle	It is usually made of china
Bed	It is comfortable	People sleep in it
Pair of trainers	They are worn on the feet	They are comfortable
Letter	It contains writing	You use it to communicate with someone
Plant	It is green and has leaves	It needs to be watered regularly
Door	It can be opened and closed	It usually has a handle
Chair	It is used for sitting on	It has four legs
Friend	Someone you like and have things in common	Someone you can play with
Ball	You can play with it	It is round and bounces
Car	It has an engine and four wheels	People go from place to place in it
Bike	It is good exercise	It has a saddle and two wheels
Sandwich	It is made of bread	It is a quick meal
Vase	It holds liquid	It is for flowers
Television	It shows programmes	You can watch it
Telephone	You can use it to talk to someone	It has buttons or a dial
Banana	It is healthy to eat	It is yellow and curve-shaped
A pair of scissors	It has two handles	It is used for cutting
Book	It can be read	It is full of stories or information
Cat	It is soft and furry and it purrs	You can stroke it

Emotions

(Unit 6 Activity 8)

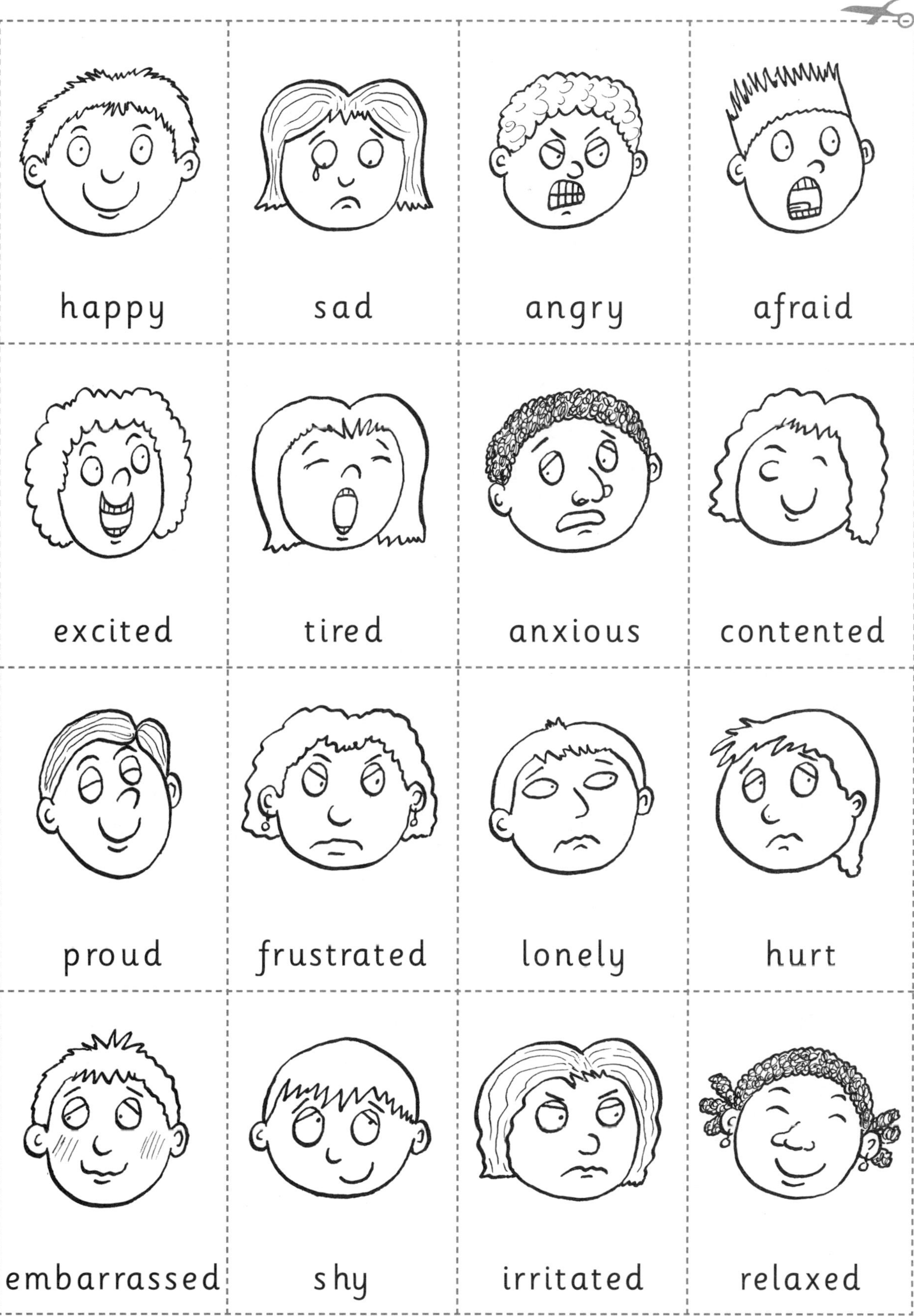

Role cards

(Unit 6 Activity 16)

Boss	Listener	Student	Sister	Leader
Peacemaker	Partner	Critic	Parent	Talker
Judge	Teacher	Dreamer	Player	Loner
Brother	Worrier	Follower	Destroyer	Decision-maker
Helper	Enemy	Guard	Maker	Carer
Doctor	Friend	Joker	Thinker	Spy

Throw a ball/Throw back

Call partner's name/Respond

Line up/Line up behind

Hold the door open/Walk through

Give a note/Read it

Smile/Smile back

Say goodbye/Walk away

Hand the phone/Talk into it

Serve dinner/Eat

Give a present/Open it

Switch on the television/Sit and watch

Knock on the door/Open it

Ask 'How are you?'/Say 'I'm fine, how are you?'

Hold out your hand, palm up/Give something

Give a compliment/Say 'Thank you'

Storyboard
(Unit 7 Activity 15)

SCENE (Number/Title)		ACTION	DIALOGUE

Six-part story
(Unit 7 Activity 16)

What is the title of the story?

What is:
The setting

The main character(s)

The problem

A helper

The solution

The outcome or ending

and	so	then
before	later	because
until	if	soon
but	just	still

Object changing emotion
(Unit 8 Activity 3)

Trying on clothing in a shop and damaging it in the process

Using a tool to make something, then injuring your finger

Opening a present but feeling disappointment when you see it

Enjoying riding your bike, then someone shouting at you for riding in a restricted area

Playing an exciting game with a friend and losing

Putting on a film to watch not realising it is frightening

Being hungry but given food you do not like to eat

Meeting up with a friend who says they have invited along someone you do not like

Appendix II

Useful Contacts

1 Fabric

All kinds of fabric can be ordered and sent by mail, including strong 100 per cent Lycra cloth in a range of primary colours.

Borovick Fabrics Ltd
16 Berwick Street
London W1F 0HP

Tel: 020 7437 2180
Web: www.borovickfabricsltd.co.uk

2 Balls

Balls of all sizes, including slow motion balls, sensory balls, heavy balls, balls that are easy to catch, as well as parachutes, streamers and tunnels.

ROMPA
Goyt Side Road
Chesterfield
Derbyshire S40 2PH

Tel: 01246 211777
Web: www.rompa.com

3 Mirrors

For single-panel mirrors as well as a very nice three-way mirror.

GALT Educational
Johnsonbrook Road
Hyde
Cheshire SK14 4QT

Tel: 08451 203005
Web: www.galt-educational.co.uk

4 Puppets

A huge selection of people, animal, fantasy and fictional character hand puppets.

Puppets by Post

Web: www.puppetsbypost.com

5 Talking Photo Album

Really nice for dressing up, character and role work. Gives grounding for imaginary play.

R-E-M
Great Western House
Langport
Somerset TA10 9BR

Tel: 01458 254700
Web: www.r-e-m.co.uk

6 A Box Full of Feelings by M Kog, J Moons, L Depondt

Has scene cards based on four basic emotions, plus masks.

Smallwood Publishing Ltd
The Old Bakery
Charlton House
Dour Street
Dover
Kent CT16 1ED

Tel: 01304 226900
Web: www.smallwood.co.uk

7 Books to support emotions work with younger children

Happiness

Some Dogs Do, Jez Alborough, Walker Books, London.
Funny!, Caroline Castle & Sam Childs, Red Fox Books, New York.
One Summer Day, Kim Lewis, Walker Books, London.

Sadness

Frog in Winter, Max Velthuijs, Andersen Press, London.
Badger's Parting Gift, Susan Varley, Picture Lions, London.

Anger

Goldilocks and the Three Bears
Little Rabbit Foo Foo, Michael Rosen, Walker Books, London.

Fear

A Dark, Dark, Tale, Ruth Brown, Puffin Books, London.
Owl Babies, Martin Waddell & Patrick Benson, Walker Books, London.

8 Combimage

A box of cards with single pictures showing different aspects of a story: characters, settings, objects.

LDA
Abbeygate House
East Road
Cambridge CB1 1DB

Tel: 0845 1204776
Web: www.LDAlearning.com

9 Picture this ... Professional V3

CD-ROM from Silver Lining Multimedia that allows you to create your own picture boards, good for making bingo boards or story cards.

Tel: 0845 6021973
Web: www.onestopeducation.co.uk

10 Boardmaker

Another useful software package for making resources, this time using Picture Communication Symbols (PCS).

Web: www.mayer-johnson.com

References

Alvarez A (1999) 'Addressing the Deficit: Developmentally Informed Psychotherapy with Passive "Undrawn" Children', Alvarez A & Reid S (eds), *Autism and Personality: Findings from the Tavistock Autism Workshop*, Routledge, London and New York, NY.

American Psychiatric Association (1994) *Diagnostic and Statistical Manual of Mental Disorders,* 4th edn, American Psychiatric Association, Washington, DC.

Axline V (1989) *Play Therapy,* Churchill Livingstone, New York, NY.

Baker S (2000) 'Learning Through Pictures', *Communication*, Spring, pp15–17.

Baron-Cohen S (1995) *Mindblindness: An Essay on Autism and Theory of Mind,* MIT Press, Cambridge, MA.

Boal A (1992) *Games for Actors and Non-Actors,* 2nd edn, Routledge, London and New York, NY.

Bogdashina O (2003) *Sensory Perceptual Issues in Autism and Asperger Syndrome,* Jessica Kingsley Publishers, London and Philadelphia, PA.

Bourgeois L (1998) *Destruction of the Father, Reconstruction of the Father: Writings and Interviews 1923-1997,* Violette Editions, London.

Brazelton TB, Koslowski B & Main M (1974) 'The Origins of Reciprocity: The Early Mother-Infant Interaction', Lewis M & Rosenblum LA (eds), *The Effect of the Infant on its Caregivers,* Wiley, Chichester.

Brody VA (1997) *The Dialogue of Touch: Developmental Play Therapy,* Jason Aronson, Northvale, NJ.

Brook P (1968) *The Empty Space,* Penguin, Harmondsworth.

Brosterman N (1997) *Inventing Kindergarten,* Harry N Abrams, New York, NY.

Bruner J & Feldman C (1993) 'Theories of Mind and the Problem of Autism', Baron-Cohen S, Tager-Flusberg H & Cohen DJ (eds), *Understanding Other Minds: Perspectives from Autism,* Oxford University Press, Oxford.

Cattanach A (1997) *Children's Stories in Play Therapy,* Jessica Kingsley Publishers, London.

Chesner A (1998) *Groupwork with Learning Disabilities: Creative Drama,* Speechmark Publishing Ltd, Brackley.

Christie P & Prevezer W (1998) *Interactive Play,* Early Years Diagnostic Centre, Ravenshead.

Christie P & Wimpory D (1986) 'Recent Research into the Development of Communicative Competence and its Implications for the Teaching of Autistic Children', *Communication* 20 (1), pp4–7.

Cicchetti D, Beeghly M & Weiss-Perry B (1994) 'Symbolic Development in Children with Down Syndrome and in Children with Autism: An Organizational, Developmental Psychopathology Perspective', Slade A & Wolff DP (eds), *Children at Play: Clinical and Developmental Approaches to Meaning and Representation,* Oxford University Press, Oxford.

Cumine V, Leach J & Stevenson G (1998) *Asperger Syndrome. A Practical Guide for Teachers,* David Fulton, London.

——— (2000) *Autism in the Early Years,* David Fulton, London.

Damasio A (2000) *The Feeling of What Happens: Body, Emotion and the Making of Consciousness,* Vintage, London.

Donaldson M (1978) *Children's Minds,* Fontana, London.

Emunah R (1994) *Acting for Real: Drama Therapy Process, Technique and Performance,* Brunner/Mazel, New York, NY.

First E (1994) 'The Leaving Game, or I'll Play You and You Play Me: The Emergence of Dramatic Role Play in 2 year olds', Slade A & Wolff DP (eds), *Children at Play: Clinical and Developmental Approaches to Meaning and Representation,* Oxford University Press, Oxford.

Gallese V (2001) 'The "Shared Manifold" Hypothesis: From Mirror Neurons to Empathy' Thompson E (ed), *Between Ourselves: Second-Person Issues in the Study of Consciousness,* Imprint Academic, Thorverton.

Gendlin ET (1978) *Focusing,* Bantam, London.

Gerland G (1996) *A Real Person: Life on the Outside,* Souvenir Press, London.

Gillberg C (2004) Keynote address, Autism Cymru International Conference, Cardiff.

Goffman E (1959) *The Presentation of Self in Everyday Life,* Doubleday, New York, NY.

Grandin T & Johnson C (2005) *Animals in Translation,* Bloomsbury, London.

Grandin T & Scariano MM (1986) *Emergence Labelled Autistic,* Warner Books, New York, NY.

Gray C (1997) *Social Stories and Comic Strip Conversations,* Speechmark Publishing, Brackley.

Hannah L (2001) *Teaching Young Children with Autistic Spectrum Disorders to Learn: A Practical Guide for Parents and Staff in Mainstream Schools and Nurseries,* National Autistic Society, London.

Hobson P (2002) *The Cradle of Thought,* Macmillan, London.

Jennings S (1986) *Creative Drama in Groupwork,* Speechmark Publishing, Brackley.

———— (1987) *Dramatherapy: Theory and Practice for Teachers and Clinicians,* Croom Helm, London and Sydney.

———— (ed) (1995) *Dramatherapy with Children and Adolescents,* Routledge, London and New York, NY.

Johnston C (1998) *House of Games: Making Theatre from Everyday Life,* Routledge, New York/Nick Hern Books, London.

Jones P (1996) *Drama as Therapy: Theatre as Living,* Routledge, London and New York, NY.

Jordan R & Powell S (1995) *Understanding and Teaching Children with Autism,* Wiley, Chichester.

Kanner L (1943) 'Autistic Disturbances of Affective Contact', *Nervous Child* 2, pp217–50.

Lahad M (1992) 'Story-making in Assessment Method for Coping with Stress', Jennings S (ed), *Dramatherapy: Theory and Practice 2,* Tavistock/Routledge, London and New York, NY.

Legler DM (1991) *Don't Take it so Literally,* ECL, Arizona, AZ.

Leslie AM (1987) 'Pretense and Representation: The Origins of "Theory of Mind"', *Psychological Review* 94 (4), pp412–26.

Leslie AM & Roth D (1993) 'What Autism Teaches Us about Metarepresentation', Baron-Cohen S, Tager-Flusberg H & Cohen DJ (eds), *Understanding Other Minds: Perspectives from Autism,* Oxford University Press, Oxford.

Moor J (2002) *Playing, Laughing and Learning with Children on the Autistic Spectrum,* Jessica Kingsley Publishers, London and Philadelphia, PA.

Mosley J (1998) *Quality Circle Time,* LDA, Cambridge.

Nind M (2000) 'Intensive Interaction and Children with Autism', Powell S (ed), *Helping Children with Autism to Learn,* David Fulton, London.

Nind M & Hewett D (1994) *Access to Communication,* David Fulton, London.

Opie I & Opie P (1959) *The Lore and Language of Schoolchildren,* Oxford University Press, Oxford.

———— (eds) (1992) *I Saw Esau: The Schoolchild's Pocket Book,* Candlewick Press, Cambridge, MA.

Piaget J (1954) *The Construction of Reality in a Child,* Basic Books, New York, NY.

Povenelli DJ & Simon BB (1998) 'Young Children's Understanding of Briefly versus extremely Delayed Images of the Self: Emergence of the Autobiographical Stance', *Developmental Psychology* 34 (1), pp188–94.

Powell S (ed) (2000) *Helping Children with Autism to Learn,* David Fulton, London.

Powell S & Jordan R (1993) 'Being Subjective about Autistic Thinking and Learning to Learn', *Educational Psychology* 13, pp359–70.

Prevezer W (2000) 'Musical Interaction and Children with Autism', Powell S (ed), *Helping Children with Autism to Learn,* David Fulton, London.

Rhode M (2001) 'The Sense of Abundance in Relation to Technique', Edwards J (ed), *Being Alive: Building on the Work of Anne Alvarez,* Brunner-Routledge, East Sussex.

Rinaldi W (1992) *The Social Use of Language Programme,* NFER-Nelson, London.

Schroeder A (1997) *Socially Speaking,* LDA, Cambridge.

Sherborne V (1990) *Developmental Movement for Children,* Cambridge University Press, Cambridge.

Spolin V (1986) *Theater Games for the Classroom: A Teacher's Handbook,* Northwestern University Press, Evanston, IL.

Stern D (1974) 'Mother and Infant at Play: The Dyadic Interaction involving Facial, Vocal and Gaze Behaviours', Lewis M & Rosenblum LA (eds), *The Effect of the Infant on its Caregiver,* Wiley, Chichester.

———— (1985) *The Interpersonal World of the Infant,* Basic Books, New York.

Taylor G (1997) 'Community Building in Schools: Developing a Circle of Friends', *Educational and Child Psychology* 14 (3), pp45–50.

Trevarthan C (2006) 'The Psychobiology of Sympathy: Infants Teach Us How Human Brains in Human Bodies Make Sense Together', Paper presented at Centre for Child Mental Health, London, 10 May 2006.

Trevarthen C, Aitken K, Papoudi D & Robarts J (1996) *Children with Autism: Diagnosis and Interventions to Meet their Needs,* 2nd edn, Jessica Kingsley Publishers, London.

Tronick EZ (1989) 'Emotions and Emotional Communication in Infants', *American Psychologist* 44 (2), pp112–19.

Vygotsky LS (1978) *Mind in Society,* Cole M, John-Steiner V, Scribner S & Souberman E (eds), Harvard University Press, Cambridge, MA.

Williams D (1992) *Nobody, Nowhere,* Corgi, London.

———— (1996) *Autism – An Inside-Out Approach,* Jessica Kingsley Publishers, London and Philadelphia, PA.

Wing L & Gould J (1979) 'Severe Impairments of Social Interaction and Associated Abnormalities in Children: Epidemiology and Classification', *Journal of Autism and Developmental Disorders* 9, pp11-29.

Wolfberg PJ (1999) *Play and Imagination in Children with Autism,* Teachers College Press, New York, NY.

World Health Organisation (1992) *International Statistical Classification of Diseases and Related Health Problems,* 10th edn, WHO, Geneva.

Index